Dynamic Psychotherapy: An Introductory Approach

Dynamic Psychotherapy: An Introductory Approach

Marc H. Hollender, M.D.
Professor of Psychiatry, Emeritus
Vanderbilt University School of Medicine
Nashville, Tennessee

Charles V. Ford, M.D.
Professor of Psychiatry
University of Alabama–Birmingham
Birmingham, Alabama

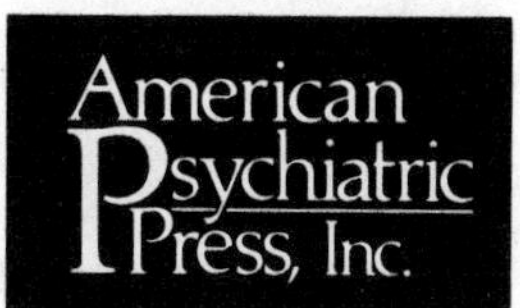

Washington, D.C.
London, England

NOTE: The contributors have worked to ensure that all information in this book concerning drug doses, schedules, and routes of administration is accurate at the time of publication and consistent with the standards set by the U.S. Food and Drug Administration and the general medical community. As medical research and practice advance, however, therapeutic standards may change. For this reason and because human and mechanical errors sometimes occur, we recommend that readers follow the advice of a physician directly involved in their care or the care of a member of their family.

Manufactured in the United States of America
91 92 93 94 5 4 3 2

American Psychiatric Press, Inc.
1400 K Street, N.W.
Washington, DC 20005

The paper used in this publication meets the minimum requirements of American National Standard for Information Sciences—Permanence of Paper for Printed Library Materials, ANSI Z39.48-1984.

Library of Congress Cataloging-in-Publication Data

Hollender, Marc H. (Marc Hale), 1916–
Dynamic psychotherapy : an introductory approach / Marc H. Hollender, Charles V. Ford.
p. cm.
Includes bibliographical references.
ISBN 0-88048-319-9
1. Psychodynamic psychotherapy. I. Ford, Charles V., 1937– II. Title.
[DNLM: 1. Psychotherapy—methods. WM 420 H737d]
RC489.P72H64 1990
616.89′14—dc20
DNLM/DLC
for Library of Congress 90-77
CIP

British Cataloguing in Publication Data

A CIP record is available from the British Library

Contents

Acknowledgments

Our thinking about dynamic psychotherapy in large measure derives from the patients we have treated and the students we have taught. Based on these experiences we have produced chapters that have been read critically by colleagues whose opinions we value. In this group were Eugene A. Kaplan, M.D.; Joseph N. DiGiacomo, M.D.; Hans H. Strupp, Ph.D.; and Howard B. Roback, Ph.D. The entire manuscript was read by two colleagues, Miles K. Crowder, M.D., and David G. Folks, M.D., and we are especially grateful to them for the time they spent and the helpful criticism they provided. Many residents read portions of the book. Those residents who contributed significantly were Frank Brown, M.D., Terri Steele, M.D., Daniel Dahl, M.D., Sarah Brown Alor, M.D., Daniel R. Garst, M.D., and Michael C. Reed, M.D.

Because our approach is that of clinicians (rather than as theoreticians), we have depended, to a considerable extent, on case reports and clinical vignettes. These we have gathered from our own practices, from the residents we supervised, and from students who took part in our seminars and classes. As we heard about patients whose treatment, good or bad, might lend itself to future teaching exercises, we stored away this information in folders simply marked, "Psychotherapy—for teaching." Unfortunately, we kept no record of who supplied the notes or when they were filed away. For this reason we cannot make appropriate individual acknowledgments. We can only acknowledge our debt and thank our trainees collectively. And this we do most sincerely.

Frederick Guggenheim, M.D., Marie Wilson Howells Professor and Chairman of the Department of Psychiatry at the University of Arkansas School for Medical Sciences, was supportive of this project and also provided constructive criticism.

Mrs. Margie Bennett and Mrs. Dana Bates (both at the University of Arkansas) and Mrs. Suzanne Flatt (at Vanderbilt University) supplied technical assistance that was invaluable. We are most appreciative of their conscientiousness and efficiency.

Finally, we would like to thank the American Psychiatric Press for their cooperation.

Preface

We have written this book for beginning and intermediate psychotherapists who wish to learn more about dynamic psychotherapy. Our emphasis throughout will be on the practical rather than the theoretical. For the most part, we will begin with the clinical situation and work from it. The area covered will encompass a wide range of psychopathology. Whenever possible, the focus will be on the here and now, from which we will try to discern the nature of the "blueprints," drawn in the past, that are shaping present-day feelings and behavior.

In planning for this book, we were stirred by our memories of *A Primer for Psychotherapists* by Kenneth Colby. That slender volume of 167 pages graced the library shelves of many beginning therapists in the decades of the 1950s and 1960s. It was popular because it was brief, it was to the point, and it offered practical advice. However, despite our fond memories of the *Primer*, we must acknowledge that it is now markedly out-of-date. It predates DSM-III-R, effective psychopharmacology, and the techniques of time-limited psychotherapy. Further, some of the advice proffered, now 40 years old, seems curiously anachronistic (such as suggesting the use of the couch for psychotherapy patients whenever possible and advising therapists who smoke to do so during therapy sessions to reduce tension).

It is our goal to provide a sound infrastructure of the principles of dynamic psychotherapy rather than to produce a "state-of-the-art" book or an encyclopedia of the various psychotherapies and techniques. It is likely that most of the ideas we espouse will be consonant with those of the majority of the educators who supervise trainees. Almost inevitably, however, there will be some who prefer an alternative approach. We would suggest that such differences of opinion may serve a valuable educational function by stimulating discussion. Certainly, we would not insist dogmatically that the approach we favor is necessarily the best or that there is only one correct way to proceed.

We have not described special therapeutic approaches to specific entities (e.g., borderline disorder or pathological narcissism). Recent innovations may be both interesting and valuable, but they are simply beyond the scope planned for our presentation. Accordingly, for more information, we recommend that the reader turn to the rich literature available on these topics.

A Reader's Guide

This volume is designed to provide a comprehensive description and detailed discussion of the dynamic psychotherapies that range from insight-oriented to supportive and from time-limited to interminable. Ideally, this book should be used to supplement individual supervision, but it can stand on its own or serve as assigned reading for a psychotherapy seminar.

The theoretical undergirding for this exposition is basically psychoanalytic, with the role of the unconscious considered central to the dynamic process. In insight-oriented psychotherapy, our understanding of the meaning of the unconscious is conveyed to the patient in interpretations; in supportive psychotherapy it is used to shape the therapist's approach; and for management it helps to determine the strategy. We have written about insight-oriented and supportive approaches as if they are sharply demarcated and clearly separated. If they ever are, it is strictly for didactic purposes. We are aware that the two approaches are almost always mixed to some extent. It is only the degree to which each approach is utilized that determines the characterization of a therapy approach as insight-oriented or supportive.

Supportive or time-limited treatment techniques are sometimes regarded as second-class therapeutic approaches. It is our contention that when appropriately applied they require technical skill equivalent to that needed for long-term insight-oriented psychotherapy and are comparably effective. We have been impressed that those therapists who are most skilled in the use of insight-oriented techniques are most capable of varying their approach for supportive psychotherapy.

Because it is very difficult to outline several ongoing processes simultaneously, we will first describe the steps involved in conducting insight-oriented psychotherapy. Then we will move on to the modifications required for time-limited therapy, supportive therapy, management techniques, and psychotherapy combined with or augmented by medication.

Issues related to psychotherapy are discussed at the approximate time they are likely to become relevant. Included are such topics as the significance of different patient referral sources, recommendations on how to set up the initial appointment, and even such practical issues as the arrangement of office furniture.

Proceeding in a stepwise progression, we will turn to the activities involved in beginning, conducting, and terminating psychotherapy. Based on an evaluation, the type of treatment to be offered is selected. If it is accepted by the patient, an agreement is reached or a "contract" is made.

Beginning with the initial phase, the nature of the relationship between the therapist and patient—realistic and transferential—is presented as being of major importance. The technical issues that are defined and discussed include interpretations, comments, questions, resistance, regression, and dream analysis. In all instances we have striven to maintain our focus on the pragmatic rather than on the arcane.

We agree with therapists, beginning with Freud, who stated that it is not possible to describe the middle phase of therapy in the same manner as it is possible to describe the opening and concluding phases. Nevertheless, we have set down guidelines to help in the selection of what we believe are the best therapeutic strategies.

Separate chapters have been devoted to a discussion of problem situations and difficult patients, how psychotherapy works, and the combination of dynamic psychotherapy and pharmacotherapy.

The case reports and clinical vignettes used in this book to illustrate major points were selected because they were especially striking and well suited to our purpose. Of course, all patient descriptions have been disguised to protect the patients' right to confidentiality.

It is not our intention to convey the impression that the material of most therapy sessions is as clearly presented and as easily understood as reflected in the brief case examples used here. This statement also holds true for the interpretation of dreams. Some dreams that are extremely difficult to decode may simply remain unanalyzed. We have made a concerted effort to avoid the use of words that essentially express value judgments. It has been our aim to describe rather than label. A word such as "mature" may have a generally accepted meaning when used to describe physical development, but when applied to human behavior it may merely express the observer's preference for a particular kind of activity.

We have made a concerted effort to avoid words for which there are no generally accepted definitions, words that superficially sound acceptable but do not withstand in-depth scrutiny. "Normal" and "neurotic" are two prime examples. Here, the problem is that educated observers do not agree on what is normal and what is neurotic, and perhaps never will.

We recommend that readers first read the book through in its entirety and then keep it handy for use as a guide when various issues arise during psychotherapy. The book is constructed as a "how-to" manual to facilitate its use as a handy reference. However, psychotherapy cannot be conducted with a "cookbook" approach. We believe that it is the richness of the varieties of human experience, the complexities of interpersonal relationships, and the unending interaction of the psychic and biological systems that make dynamic psychotherapy an art as well as a craft and a science.

1

Psychotherapy: What, When, and Why?

Is psychotherapy merely the process of buying a friend? If not, how does it differ from other personal relationships? Does it work, and if so, how? When and for what reasons should a person seek psychotherapy?

We shall attempt to offer beginning answers to these oft-asked questions in this introductory chapter while keeping in mind that further and more complete elucidation is still being provided by psychotherapy research.

Definition

Psychotherapy has been loosely defined as the systematic use of a human relationship for therapeutic purposes—to effect enduring changes in the patient's thinking, feelings, and behavior (Strupp 1986). Six features have been identified as being common to all psychotherapies: 1) an intense, emotionally charged, confiding relationship with a helping person; 2) a rationale, which includes an explanation of the cause of the patient's distress and a method for relieving it; 3) provision of new information concerning the nature and sources of the patient's problems and possible ways of dealing with them; 4) strengthening the patient's expectations of help through the personal qualities and status of the therapist; 5) provision of success experiences that heighten hope and enhance a sense of mastery; and 6) facilitation of emotional arousal, which seems to be a prerequisite to attitudinal and behavioral changes (Frank 1971).

In defining a particular type of psychotherapy, it is necessary to describe several features because no single feature is "diagnostic." Often more than one name is given to a type of psychotherapy, each name being derived from distinctive features. For example, an insight-oriented approach might also be referred to as psychoanalytic, uncovering, or reconstructive psychotherapy.

The common thread running through the psychotherapies we shall describe in this book is the pursuit and use of an understanding of the unconscious dimension. This information may be imparted to the patient or it may simply shape the therapist's approach. Either way it is the pivotal feature that makes the process dynamic.

In some respects, psychotherapy resembles a medical procedure, and in other respects it resembles an educational endeavor. Like medicine it is designed to relieve distress, which is usually experienced as anxiety, depression, or psychosomatic symptoms.

Psychotherapy is similar to education, but the learning is of a personal nature. Bellak (1977) stated that psychotherapy involves unlearning, learning, and relearning. The patient must learn how to undo old maladaptive patterns (unlearning), develop new and more effective coping mechanisms (learning or "working through"), and then reinforcing these new patterns of behavior (relearning) by repetition. In addition to conveying information about patterns of thinking, feeling, and behavior, the therapist—like a good teacher—exerts a profound effect by his or her impact as a person (learning by identification with the therapist).

Cultural Context

Despite striking differences, all forms of psychotherapy share certain basic conditions. There is a therapist who, like the healer of old, is reputed to possess the power to help others, and there is the patient who turns to the therapist seeking help. All therapies attempt to influence the patient in three ways—cognitively, emotionally, and behaviorally—but some emphasize one way much more than the other two (Tseng and McDermott 1975; Karasu 1986).

In discussing the cultural orientation, Frank (1959) stated,

> The belief of members of a culture as to what constitutes illness and its treatment are formed and supported by generally held cultural attitudes. A member of a particular society can regard himself as having an emotional illness—for which the proper treatment is psychotherapy—only if his society recognizes the existence of such illnesses and sanctions psychotherapy as the appropriate treatment for them.

Yet, the goals of psychotherapy are to increase patients' comfort and functioning and not specifically to help them "adjust" to society.

Who Needs and Who Can Benefit from Psychotherapy?

The question of who might benefit from psychotherapy is often debated. At times it is answered in a global way: that all persons might benefit from psychotherapy by gaining greater insight into themselves and learning more about how to relate to others. Despite the obvious appeal of such an all-inclusive statement, it is not correct. Persons who function well can spend their time in better ways than in a narcissistic preoccupation with themselves. Also, as will be discussed below, for some persons psychotherapy may have a deleterious effect. For others, psychotherapy may be an elective procedure. They may experience areas of discomfort in their lives or have symptoms that prevent them from being as effective as they might be in various social, educational, or interpersonal situations. Yet, they manage, as most of us do, to fulfill the basic needs of life. For them psychotherapy can be regarded as a luxury, something desirable if possible, but not mandatory. An analogy might be drawn to plastic surgery in that some procedures, carrying relatively little risk, might enhance one's appearance but are optional. (Again, similar to the situation with plastic surgery, the following question might appropriately be asked: If this is a luxury, who should bear the expense? Should it be an insurance company or other third-party payers or should it be reserved for those who wish to spend their discretionary resources in this manner?)

Another group, for whom treatment is clearly indicated, is comprised of persons whose symptoms are severe enough to significantly impair their ability to function in their occupations or to manage day-to-day responsibilities as marital partners, parents, or members of the community. They need help, much as does any person who has a medical illness. For them the question is: Is psychotherapy the most efficacious treatment or are there alternative approaches that would work as well or better? Until fairly recently, with the advent of psychotropic medications, the answer was that psychotherapy was the best we had to offer. In retrospect, it appears to have provided relatively little effect on the prognosis of disorders such as schizophrenia or mania. However, even for those disorders, psychotherapy did supply some comfort and hope and therefore provided some therapeutic benefit.

With the excitement resulting from the introduction of psychotropic medications, some thought psychotherapy might well be superseded. However, more recently, several controlled studies (Elkin et al. 1989; Conte et al. 1986; Woody et al. 1987; Klerman et al. 1987) indicate that psychotherapy, either alone or combined with psychotropic medications, when judiciously administered for specific disorders, is a potent and effective treatment modality.

When Is Psychotherapy Sought?

Patients generally seek help when a major change in their lives causes significant discomfort. Life stressors may trigger an underlying psychiatric disorder (e.g., major depression), may produce dysphoric emotions related to problems of adjustment (e.g., separation anxiety associated with divorce), may produce symptoms that interfere with effective coping mechanisms and/or interpersonal relationships (e.g., irritability associated with occupational pressures), or the apparent stressors may themselves be the product of an underlying psychiatric disorder and/or of personality characteristics (e.g., business failures caused by hypomania, or being discharged from a job because of chronic tardiness and procrastination).

As a rule, persons seek psychotherapy at a time of stress. They may have long toyed with the notion, but it is the acute life event that finally tips the scale and prompts them to call for an appointment with a therapist. It is then, because of acute discomfort and the wish for relief, that the patient's motivation appears to be the greatest.

Another time that patients may be especially receptive to engaging in psychotherapy is when they are physically ill. Wahl (1972) related this phenomenon to the regression that occurs during bouts of illness and to the fact that some rigid defenses become less prominent. At such times it may be possible to establish a close, positive relationship with a patient that continues after the physical symptoms remit.

Psychotherapy for Better or Worse

Since psychotherapy is indeed potent and effective when used appropriately, much like any potent and effective medication, it can have adverse effects when used improperly. The provocative book, *Psychotherapy for Better or Worse*, by Strupp et al. (1977) is based on this premise. It should be kept in mind, before beginning, that psychotherapy is a complex endeavor and is not to be undertaken casually. When patients who are not really candidates for this approach are forced into a preshaped mold, the result is likely to be unfortunate.

At times psychotherapy may serve the psychological needs of the therapist more than those of the patient. For example, persons who need to be controlling, or to gain a sense of importance or power, may be attracted to a profession in which patients turn to them asking for help. Here is a clinical example:

> *A man being evaluated for psychotherapy expressed doubts that he would be helped, based on a previous experience with a therapist. When questioned about this experience, he replied, "She [the therapist] was too busy telling me what to do to try and find out what was wrong with me."*

Other types of unfortunate and antitherapeutic encounters that have been observed involve therapists who act out their unconscious sadistic or competitive impulses by continually criticizing patients, finding fault, and possibly even passing moral judgment. Another type of undesirable encounter occurs when therapists use therapy as a setting for self-glorification. They do so by encouraging patients to tell them how brilliant, powerful, insightful, or attractive they are. Among the most exploitative and reprehensible types of behavior in which a therapist might engage are those involving a sexual relationship. Not only does such behavior have a deleterious effect in the present, but it is likely to interfere with the patient's ability to have a trusting therapeutic relationship in the future (Webb 1988).

To be effective, therapists should have the capacity for psychological insightfulness that includes self-criticism. The feelings of the therapist and therapeutic errors cannot be completely separated from this imperfect process. In the past, it was thought that therapists would have to undergo a personal analysis to be effective. Certainly at times such an experience would be helpful. However, it is not always necessary or practical. Moreover, a personal analysis is no guarantee that countertransference problems or acting out by a therapist will not occur. Yet, as noted previously, introspection and a capacity for self-criticism are essential if the probability of a favorable outcome is to be appreciably greater than that of an unfavorable one.

How Does Psychotherapy Work?

First, the relationship with the therapist (who may be seen as a benign but powerful healing authority) may have a positive effect in reducing anxiety and encouraging hope and optimism. Second, the therapist, of necessity, becomes a part of the patient's social support system and often has an ameliorating effect on both psychic and physiologic symptoms.

Perhaps the most important effect of psychotherapy, however, is educational. The word educational is used here in its broadest sense. Stated differently, the patient learns new behavioral patterns, sometimes ways to respond physiologically and physically, and most importantly, ways to think about life experiences as well as techniques that can be used to solve problems in the future (Strupp 1969).

Through gaining insight, which is an educational process, it can be discerned how old patterns were created—and how unconscious forces shaped unwanted behavior. As a result of greater insight into these unconscious processes (making the unconscious, conscious), the number of choices is increased. It should be emphasized, however, that insight per se does not bring about change. (For a detailed discussion of how therapy works, see Chapter 8.)

Summary

Psychotherapy is the systematic use of an interpersonal relationship to effect cognitive, affective, and behavioral changes in patients. These changes occur primarily through a "learning" process. Because psychotherapy is a potent modality, it has the capacity for adverse as well as therapeutic effects. Psychotherapy is not a universal panacea; there are specific indications. Persons who will benefit from psychotherapy tend to be most receptive at times of psychological or physiological crises in their lives.

2

The Initial Contact

The relationship between patient and therapist is shaped in part even before their initial meeting. In this chapter this will be shown as we consider the sources of referral, issues concerned with making the initial appointment, and the physical facility in which the patient is seen. We will also make some general comments about the quality of the "social" interaction between therapist and patient.

Sources of Referral

Patients are referred by a variety of sources, including self-referral. Each source of referral requires a somewhat different approach, since the source can determine the attitude the potential patient will have toward the process of psychotherapy and the proposed therapist.

The Self-Referred Patient

Some patients who are self-referred are good prospects for psychotherapy. The fact that they have taken the initiative in making the appointment suggests that they are motivated for change and recognize some individual responsibility for their own care. Among the "best" of these patients are those who have been given the name of the therapist by a friend previously or currently in treatment with the therapist. The friend probably made the recommendation because of warm and positive feelings toward his or her own therapy. Consequently, the prospective patient is likely to arrive with an optimistic and even enthusiastic attitude. Additionally, the friend may have described the process of therapy itself, what to expect in terms of the mechanics (e.g., fees, hours, policies) as well as the style of treatment itself. Such information, of course, can be a two-edged sword, since the prospective patient's expectations may be somewhat different from what would be appropriate for his or her individual needs.

The therapist's name may also have been obtained from a person seen in a professional relationship, for example, a physician or a clergyman. These professionals have varying amounts of information about the process of therapy and/or the personal characteristics and techniques of a particular therapist. Often the therapist is selected by reputation only and, therefore, the prospective patient has relatively little information except that the therapist is supposed to be "good." Information provided to the prospective patient may be basically incorrect due to misunderstandings about the nature of psychotherapy on the part of the person making the referral. In extreme instances, impossible promises may be made about what therapy will accomplish. One man was referred by his internist with the goal of "helping him get married" in order to "cure" his homosexual fantasies.

The self-referred patient may have obtained the name of the therapist from a completely random source, for example, from a telephone listing, local medical society, or mental health association. Although some of these patients do prove to be able to work constructively in psychotherapy, many of them do not. For example, they may be incipiently psychotic or in acute legal difficulty and blindly searching for some type of assistance. These prospective patients can be screened by some of the techniques described in this chapter.

The Direct Referral

It is not unusual for a physician or other professional to attempt to make a direct appointment for a patient, thereby bypassing the need for the prospective patient to take the initiative. This procedure, commonplace for medical referrals, has troubled psychiatrists who, like other specialists, have rules and routines that sometimes are followed blindly and defended like sacred cows (Hollender 1979). According to one such rule, prospective patients should be required to call for their own appointments. The phone call is regarded as a test of motivation for treatment, but it should be asked if motivation must be tested before an evaluation has been completed.

If the concern is that patients are more likely to miss appointments when they have not participated in scheduling them, two possible approaches might be taken. The first is to request that the referring physician ask the patient to call a certain number of days before the appointment to confirm that it will be kept. The other is to have the receptionist in the therapist's own office call the patient as a reminder.

If the first appointment is kept, no matter who has made it, an evaluation can be conducted and appropriate treatment offered. Then, if it is desirable to assess the motivation of a potential candidate for psychotherapy, the therapist might say, "Please consider the treatment plan I have recommended. If you wish to discuss it further or if you wish to begin treatment, call me within a week."

Another form of direct referral involves a therapist referring a patient who was seen in an inpatient setting or an emergency room to himself or herself for outpatient psychotherapy. This particular situation is most likely to be encountered by psychiatric residents whose initial contact with patients may be in an acute-care setting. The advantages are obvious; the therapist has some information about the patient, and the patient, having met the therapist, has established a beginning relationship. The disadvantage is that frequently the needs of the patient in the acute-care setting were such that the therapist acted in a far more directive manner than may be desirable for psychotherapy, and it is often difficult for the patient to accept a change in the style of the relationship.

The Clinic Patient

Patients referred to an outpatient psychiatry or psychology clinic face a somewhat different situation. Clinics, by their nature, tend to be impersonal. The patient has little idea of what to expect, and the assignment to a therapist, who will conduct an evaluation, is often random. Because the therapist has not been chosen specifically by the patient, there may be more difficulty in establishing rapport. Also, it is not uncommon in clinics for one person to conduct the evaluation and another person the treatment. During the evaluation (one to three interviews), the patient may develop positive feelings toward the person conducting the evaluation and as a result there is a sense of rejection when a referral is made to another therapist. Thus, therapy may start with two strikes against it: a therapist not chosen by the patient and a sense of being rejected by the previous therapist. These feelings can be mollified to an extent if the patient is aware of them and encouragement to talk about them. Even better, the clinic routine should be arranged so that shuffling from one therapist to another is avoided.

Other Sources of Referral

Some referrals for psychotherapy may involve some degree of coercion, and although these situations do not necessarily imply a poor prognosis, there may be a significant problem with motivation. When psychotherapy has been mandated as a condition of probation, the patient may not see the need for change. In addition there may be resentment of demands made on both time and money. Because of this, therapy may be regarded as a punishment rather than as a source of help.

Some degree of coercion also exists when an employer requires or strongly hints that therapy designed to bring about a change is required as a condition for continued employment. Such a request may be ambivalently regarded if it is recognized that the employer sincerely wishes to help rather than discharge the person. A similar situation arises when insurance companies or government agencies demand some type of psychiatric evaluation and/or psychotherapy as a requirement for continued insurance benefits, disability payments, or welfare checks.

Significant numbers of persons seek psychotherapy as a condition imposed by another person for continuing a relationship. For example, a marital partner may say, "If you don't 'get help,' I will leave and divorce you."

A similar situation arises when a physician says (or implies) to a patient, "I can no longer continue to treat you, and will not have you in my medical practice if you do not see a psychiatrist (or psychologist)." Persons who apply for treatment under such circumstances often wish only to appease the other party and are not truly seeking help.

When the Prospective Patient Calls to Make the Initial Appointment

As a general rule, if the prospective patient does call to make an appointment, the call should be taken (or returned) personally by the therapist, rather than by a secretary, assistant, or clerk. During the initial telephone contact the therapist should ascertain, if possible, the nature of the referral source and the degree of urgency of the problem. This type of information generally can be obtained in two or three minutes and helps to screen inappropriate referrals.

Persons who call to request an appointment, or who call because they are considering doing so, may ask one or several questions. The questions include:

- What are the fees?
- What is the therapist's (theoretical) orientation? What therapeutic techniques does the therapist use?
- What is the nature of the therapist's professional qualifications?
- How old is the therapist?

In terms of theoretical orientation, a more specific question might be:

- Is the therapist a psychoanalyst? And if the response is positive, is the therapist a Freudian or a member of another school?

In terms of therapeutic technique, more specific questions might be:

- Does the therapist prescribe medication?
- Does the therapist use hypnosis?

Some persons are intent on finding a hypnotist, and if the therapist states that he or she does not use hypnosis, no appointment is scheduled and the contact is terminated.

In terms of qualifications, when the therapist is assigned, the prospective patient may inquire if the therapist is a psychiatrist, psychologist, or social worker.

As a rule of thumb in deciding which questions to answer, respond directly to those questions that are impersonal enough to be answered by the information usually supplied in *Who's Who* volumes or in standard professional directories.

It is not unusual to be asked a question of a somewhat personal nature, usually related to religious beliefs or affiliations. A prospective patient may ask:

- Do you accept Jesus as your savior?
- Are you a born-again Christian?
- Are you Jewish?

The therapist may counter by inquiring how the prospective patient thinks religious issues will affect treatment. Or the therapist may state that he or she has had considerable experience in treating members of various faiths and is comfortable in doing so. If the prospective patient remains unsatisfied, the contact will usually be terminated at this point.

How much information, and of what type, the patient is entitled to receive remains an open issue. We have merely expressed our viewpoint. Other therapists may draw the line at a different point. They may be willing to answer questions about religion but regard questions pertaining to the details of training and professional affiliations as personal.

Assuming that the previous discussions have resulted in the mutual desire to arrange an appointment for an evaluation, the therapist should suggest a time. As a general rule, it should be within two weeks. A significantly later appointment suggests that the therapist may be too busy to tend to the needs of the patient or is disinterested. A distant appointment time may also fail to take into account the degree of patient distress. Occasionally special or emergency appointments may be arranged outside usual practice hours. It should be made clear to the patient that such times are special and that, if therapy is proposed, future appointments will be scheduled during the therapist's normal office hours.

The therapist must be cautious about making "special appointments," in that manipulative patients often request unusual consideration. Negotiations over the scheduling of the initial appointment may represent the first effort of the manipulative patient to set the tone of the relationship.

The psychiatric outpatient clinic may create special circumstances. Not infrequently the patient has been given an arbitrary appointment time and there has been little or no consideration given to the appropriateness of the referral. Consequently, both patient and therapist may view this "assignment" with less than enthusiasm. The therapist must be aware of the nature of this process and make special efforts to establish rapport.

Often the patient will have many questions because of lack of prior information concerning the therapist or clinic. Such questions are appropriate and should not be dealt with defensively. What are the professional qualifications of the therapist? Is the therapist in training? If so, how long will the therapist be in the clinic before completing training? Is there supervision? To what degree is such supervision confidential? Will any special demands be made on the patient as a condition of providing treatment (e.g., tape recording or videotaping of the therapy sessions)?

The Unspoken Questions

Many questions, as indicated in this chapter, are raised directly by patients. However, there may still be unspoken questions that might readily be inferred. For example, one prospective patient, during an evaluation at a university psychiatric clinic, recounted her experiences at a dental school clinic. She explained that she was kept waiting for an extended period before being seen by a dental student who repeatedly left her to confer with an instructor. After spending an entire afternoon at the clinic, she was informed that the procedure she required could not be completed that day and she would have to return in two weeks.

This patient's unspoken questions are transparent. Would she be treated with respect in regard to time? Would her therapist be a student supervised by a faculty member? Would the clinic see to it that necessary procedures be finished without undue delay?

The patient was told that she obviously was concerned about the nature of the psychiatric clinic's operation, and she was provided with a description of it. She was informed that the therapists were trainees supervised by faculty members, that times were arranged with consideration given to the schedules of both therapist and patient, and that although results from therapy could not be guaranteed she could be assured of receiving continuing care.

The Physical Setting

The setting in which patients are seen conveys considerable information about the therapist and the other persons working with the therapist.

The location of the office may take on different meanings to different patients. Lewin (1965) stated, "If it is in a medical building, it can connote respectability, but it also may imply cold, clinical detachment. A setting in an apartment building or private dwelling may arouse suspicion of seduction or quackery, but also may suggest privacy, warmth, and personal attention."

The waiting room, in both a private office and a clinic setting, should afford as much privacy as possible. Rather than require the patients to sit in a circle and stare at each other, it is preferable, in large waiting areas, for the space to be subdivided either by room dividers or the arrangement of furniture. Magazines should be current. As Lewin (1965) stated, "Current magazine issues suggest that the doctor is considerate of his patients; lack of current issues implies indifference, contempt (the old ones are good enough), carelessness, or perhaps that the doctor is a slow reader." The magazines chosen often convey a subtle message about what the therapist reads or what the patient should read (e.g., *Architectural Digest* versus *People*). In recent years, there has been an unfortunate trend toward having the receptionist blocked off by a glass wall so that the only way to talk with him or her is through a window that looks strikingly like that of a bank teller.

An ideal arrangement for a private psychiatric consultation suite consists of a small waiting room, with or without a receptionist, from which there is an entrance into the consultation room. The consultation room has a second exit by which patients can leave without being seen by persons in the waiting room. It also makes it possible for the therapist to leave briefly without going through the waiting room (Figure 1). Unfortunately, this "ideal" arrangement is not often feasible.

Regardless of the layout, the essential requirement for the consultation suite is privacy. It must be designed so that what is said is not heard outside the office. Neither the receptionist nor any person in the waiting room should be able to hear even muffled

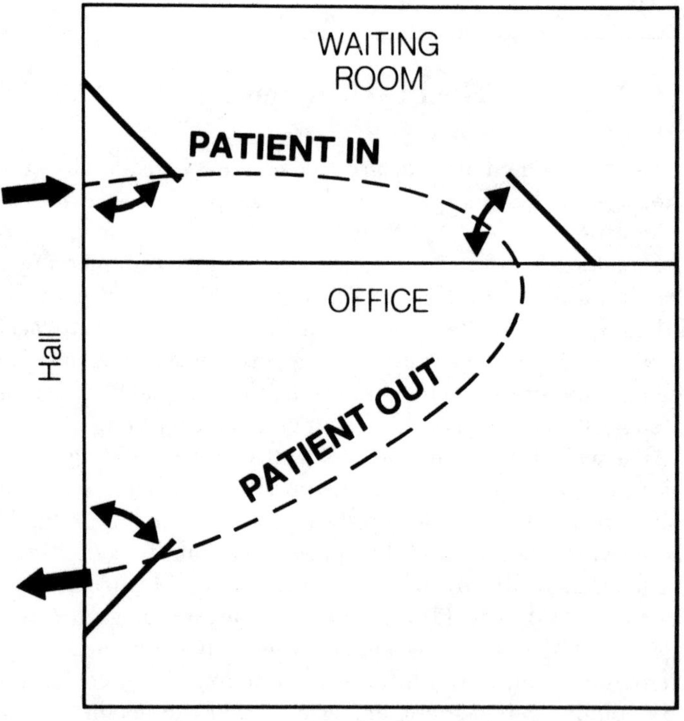

Figure 1. Ideal patient flow pattern in the therapist's office.

conversation. To ensure that nothing will be overheard, double doors and/or a music system are often used.

Experience has shown that a comfortable seating arrangement for the initial appointment is one in which the therapist sits at a desk and the prospective patient sits next to the desk (Figure 2). This provides for a professional interchange, and some notes can be made and an evaluation conducted. Once the process of therapy has begun, it is generally more comfortable for both therapist and patient to move away from the desk to other chairs in the office. The chairs (and possibly a sofa) should be arranged so that each person can look at the other without the need to stare (Figure 2).

An alternative seating arrangement is to have two chairs placed so that therapist and patient face each other but at a slight angle. The distance between the therapist and patient should be the customary conversational distance. (This distance will vary from one culture to another.) A clipboard will serve for note

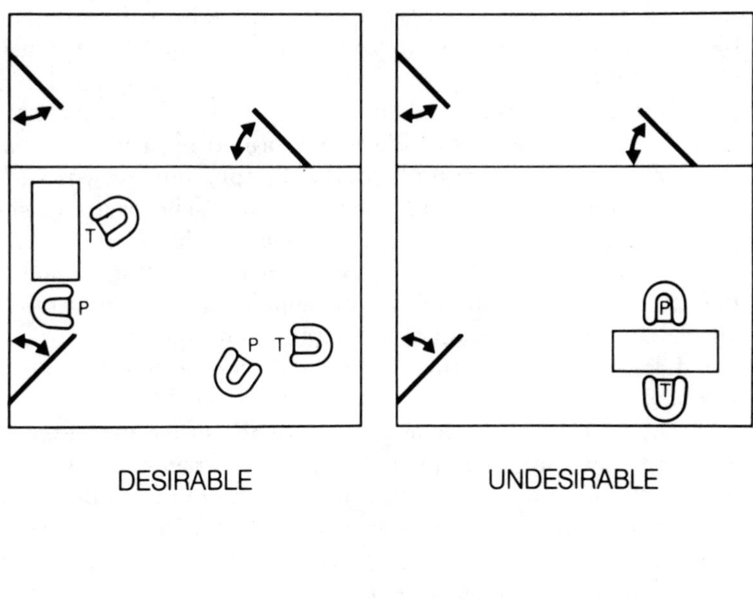

Figure 2. Arrangement of furniture in the therapist's office.

taking, and when not in use, it can be placed on a table beside the therapist's chair.

Some patients will move their chair closer to the therapist. Doing so may be in keeping with culturally determined spacing, or it may have significant psychological meaning. At the outset of therapy the reasons for the patient's move may be apparent to the therapist, but it seldom is appropriate to offer an interpretation at that time.

It is usually undesirable to have the furniture arranged for psychotherapy so that the patient is looking across a desk at the therapist. This arrangement, often used in the traditional doctor-patient relationship, is not appropriate for insight-oriented psychotherapy because it places the therapist at a distance and in an authoritarian position. However, it may sometimes be appropriate for supportive psychotherapy, when a paranoid patient needs to keep a "safe" distance and maintain an emotional wall between himself or herself and the therapist.

In general, the arrangement and decor of the office reflect the personality and personal taste of the therapist. All items say something about the therapist. That is particularly true for personal effects such as photographs and framed certificates. The therapist also should be aware of the message conveyed by such items as Bibles or souvenirs.

One psychiatrist, who had been in practice for about three years, decided to have his office redecorated by a professional interior decorator. The result was a lavish suite complete with such items as gilded mirrors and swag draperies. The psychiatrist's patients made numerous pointed comments to the effect that "no wonder the fees are so high," and long-term patients complained that the decorating did not fit the personality of the therapist they knew. After a short period of time, and at considerable expense, the therapist had his office completely redecorated in a more subdued style.

Other seemingly minor features of the office may exert a greater effect than is immediately obvious. For example, one beginning therapist decided that it would be more comfortable, for both him and his patients, if there was a coffee pot available on a small table in his office so that they could drink coffee during therapy hours. It became evident, over a period of several months, that there was a tendency for patients to attempt to use the therapy hours as "social gatherings." The therapist discovered that when the coffee pot was removed it was easier for him to maintain a professional relationship and to keep patients at the tasks of psychotherapy rather than engaged in a social interchange.

Social Conventions

Socially appropriate manners and customs convey a sense of respect for the patient. One should introduce oneself using one's name and that of the patient with the appropriate titles. For example, "Good morning, Miss Smith. I am Dr. Joseph Jones." Early in the psychotherapeutic relationship the use of first names, especially with elderly or minority race patients, conveys a sense of disrespect and/or condescension. The exception might be the use of first names with adolescents or young adults. Maintaining the appropriate social graces does not imply, however, that the situation should be converted from a professional relationship into a social interaction. For example, it is not appropriate to hold the patient's coat routinely at the end of the hour.

In our society it is customary to shake hands at the point of introduction and at the end of the first meeting but not usually thereafter. (Exceptions in supportive therapy will be discussed later.)

The current attitude about smoking favors the rights of nonsmokers. Accordingly, the therapist should not smoke in the office area or permit others to smoke there. The absence of ashtrays in the therapist's office should send a clear message. If, however, it is not adequate, a no smoking sign should be placed in the waiting room.

Getting Started

After being seated for the first appointment, the therapist can state what he or she knows about the patient: a brief recounting of what has been conveyed to the therapist by the referring source and/or the telephone conversation with the patient when setting the appointment time. Such an approach helps to clarify any misunderstandings that might have arisen.

Summary

To some degree the relationship between patient and therapist is shaped by various circumstances before therapy starts. The referral source, the appointment procedure, and the physical setting all influence the patient's expectations and fantasies, as well as the relationship. When the patient is seen in a clinic setting, there is an increased need to recognize, and respond to, certain impersonal procedures which may make it more difficult to establish rapport. Social conventions, either in their observance or neglect, may also subtly carry messages which require attention.

3

The Selection Process

As mentioned at the conclusion of Chapter 2, the initial comments to the patient should serve to clarify the reason for the consultation and to review information that had previously been provided by the patient and/or referring professional person. If it is confirmed that the information is accurate and if there are no major changes in the reason for the consultation, the therapist should proceed by asking one or more open-ended questions, preferably about something in the here-and-now. These questions should be couched in general terms so that the patient can respond spontaneously with whatever is on his or her mind and thus provide information about areas of discomfort. Examples of such open-ended questions would be, "Tell me more about why you are here" or "You told me on the telephone that you were feeling depressed. Please tell me more about how you feel."

Once the patient starts to talk, he or she should not be interrupted for at least five to 10 minutes. This allows for a spontaneous exposition of the problems. To ask questions sooner focuses on one area and away from others. At this juncture a panoramic view is needed; the detailed exploration of a particular part of the landscape can wait until later.

In regard to further questions and the theme of the interview, the therapist should stay with the initial complaint and/or problem until it has been fully explored and understood. In other words, much as an obstetrician might say, the presenting part must be delivered first. It is likely that during the evaluation, the therapist will have different ideas from the patient about what the problems actually are. However, it is poor technique, and may significantly interfere with rapport, to jump in with such ideas prematurely.

With the patient who answers even general questions with few words, it may be necessary to ask multiple questions. Doing so is preferable to enduring long silences, and the anxiety that they may engender, at this early stage of the evaluation.

The Diagnosis

Today, with the availability of new medications and with specific and nonspecific indications for their use and with the availability of several types of psychotherapy, the first question is: What is the diagnosis? To reach a working diagnosis, our approach should be both descriptive and dynamic. (Now, as in the past, the examination of the patient should include diagnostic studies for medical disorders that may present with symptoms suggestive of a psychiatric disorder.)

When evaluating the patient for therapy, it is advisable to establish a diagnosis based on the diagnostic criteria presented in the *Diagnostic and Statistical Manual of Mental Disorders*, Third Edition, Revised (DSM-III-R; American Psychiatric Association 1987). The reasons for this include medical-legal considerations as well as good medical practice. For example, some DSM-III-R diagnoses (such as major depression) call for the use of certain accepted treatment modalities. When one deviates from these standard treatment approaches, there should be a clear explanation as to the rationale. It is no longer acceptable to treat disorders such as panic attacks by psychotherapy alone unless there are unusual and compelling reasons to do so (Ballenger 1986).

However important the precise DSM-III-R diagnosis may be, it is not sufficient in itself to estimate the patient's ability to work in psychotherapy or to determine which form of treatment to recommend. Therefore, one should proceed with an evaluation that takes into account far more than diagnostic criteria.

We view with concern the increasing use of structured diagnostic interviews and evaluations that are focused only on eliciting symptoms. The current generation of psychiatric residents often seems to believe that diagnosis consists of fitting the patient to the specified criteria in DSM-III-R. Their evaluations then consist of a large number of symptom-oriented questions (e.g., Do you awake early in the morning?) that can be answered yes or no. The richness and complexity of the human experience are lost in this diagnostic reductionism as are opportunities to empathize with and therapeutically address the pain of "neurotic suffering."

Pertinent to this subject are the comments of Reiser (1988), who found it difficult to obtain a "satisfactory image and idea of the patient and his or her life situation . . . when [the residents'] approach and mind set in the interviews were astoundingly nonpsychological."

Reiser added,

> Once they [the residents] had done the DSM-III "inventory" and had identified target symptoms for pharmacotherapy, the diagnostic workup and meaningful communication stopped. Worse than that . . . so did the residents' curiosity about the patient as a person . . . even to the point where often there was no answer to such basic questions as why the patient came for treatment at this time and what seemed to be worrying him or her. Most of these residents could and would have learned more about a stranger who was sitting next to them for an hour on an airplane trip than they had learned in these formal psychiatric interviews.

We are essentially in agreement with Karasu (1980), who stated,

> Not only do few patients really fit DSM-III categories, but often this expedient but clinically limited method of assessing illness offers little of practical psychotherapeutic value. Psychotherapy-oriented diagnosis and assessment in a more constructive sense attempt to empathetically portray the patient and his inner world, his strengths as well as weaknesses, his capacities for health as well as illness. Throughout the therapeutic process, therefore, the therapist reexplores and refines his diagnosis by carefully observing the patient's interactions, his relationship to himself and others, his adaptability and accessibility for particular therapeutic interventions.

How to listen is important enough to merit some additional comments. Listening involves more than simply hearing what is said; it requires concentration and comprehension. To listen constructively, the therapist must focus on what is being said, not on the next question he or she will ask the patient. Focusing on the next question, which might be described as verbal "tailgating," should be avoided. The therapist should usually avoid interrupting the patient and appearing uninterested in what is being said. Becoming a good listener may require practice. Further, the advice of Henderson (1935) is well taken here: First, the physician should listen to what the patient wishes to say; then, to what the patient knows but does not wish to say because of shame or embarrassment; and finally, to what the patient cannot say because it is unconscious. Therapists should recognize the challenge in understanding the patient's communication: to make the "diagnosis" or fathom the meaning of unconscious messages. To meet this challenge, the therapist must function somewhat like a detective. He or she is called on to rule in or rule out certain possibilities using the power of reasoning and the pursuit of meaning. We hope to bring to life this process which remains the special province of the psychotherapist.

In a diagnostic interview, what is not said is often as important as what is said. For example, in the evaluation of one young man, an hour was spent discussing his work and his relationship with his parents and his daughter. Interestingly, and very significantly, throughout the entire hour no mention was made of his wife. It was not surprising to learn during therapy that the relationship with his wife was full of conflict.

It is important to note that information is obtained not only from the content of the patient's verbal productions, but also through nonverbal communications. The following vignette illustrates the information that may be gathered from nonverbal clues.

> *Mrs. D complained of lack of energy, of often being on the verge of tears, of early morning awakening, and of considerable weight loss. Her wan and sad expression, like her complaints, suggested profound depression. But other features were incongruent. Blue eye-shadow had been carefully applied and so had lipstick. Her clothing was neat and she wore a string of beads. The appearance that had at first suggested depression seemed more likely to be due to sedating drugs. An occasional slight slurring of speech favored that conclusion. In response to questioning the patient acknowledged that she took a large amount daily of a drug that had once been prescribed for her.*

The following issues are important in conducting an evaluation. They should not be regarded, however, as a checklist, nor should the information be obtained by slavish adherence to an interview outline. As a matter of fact, any effort to rigidly structure the interview may prevent emergence of essential clinical material that would evolve with the use of a more unstructured technique. Still, by the time that a careful evaluation has been completed, the therapist should be able to address each of the general issues considered below.

Why Is the Patient Seeking Treatment at This Time?

After gathering some information about the present complaint, an effort should be made to discern what was the event that tipped the scale and prompted the seeking of help. Rarely is chronicity responsible; almost always a specific event mobilizes the patient (or someone close to the patient) to telephone for an appointment. If it was someone other than the patient who made the call, how did the patient feel about it? If the patient comes at a relative's behest or even as a condition of parole, it does not necessarily mean that real motivation to obtain help is lacking. On the other hand, a person may come on his or her own but only to placate another person. In such an instance what superficially appears to be involvement is likely to be a sham, merely a process of going through the motions.

At times the patient has a hidden agenda. An example of this is the case of a man who sought psychiatric treatment when he was in the process of litigation in a personal injury suit. It developed that he perceived psychiatric treatment as providing additional evidence of the extent of "injury" that he had sustained. It was his notion that seeing a psychiatrist would result in a larger settlement.

The Number of Sessions for Assessment

A striking difference may be noted in how much more open and candid a patient is at the second interview than he or she was at the first interview. This change is striking but not surprising. At the initial visit there is the task of adjusting to a strange setting and a new person in addition to coping with feelings about seeking psychiatric help, perhaps for the first time. In contrast, the patient arrives at the second visit with some understanding of what to expect and how to behave.

Comments made and questions raised by the interviewer may have given the patient much to think about in the days between sessions. An interpretation made in the initial session might serve as a trial balloon, providing a reading on how introspective and psychologically minded the patient can be. This reading might come in the form of an immediate response or in statements made during the following hour.

Although an evaluation can sometimes be completed in a single session, there are many instances in which additional information obtained in a second or even a third interview is important, if not indispensable, in determining the appropriate therapy to recommend.

There comes a time, usually during the second interview, when history-taking should stop if it has not already and certain immediate issues should be addressed. These issues include: Why does the patient come for help *now* ? What *kind* of help (symptom relief or character change) does the patient seek? What is the patient's picture of treatment? These are the questions that should be answered, or at least partially answered, before making recommendations and reaching an agreement on how to proceed.

Reasons for Seeking Treatment

Among the host of reasons for seeking outpatient (office or clinic) care, uncomfortable or troublesome symptoms such as anxiety or depression are high on the list. Other reasons for consulting a therapist are much less common, and some are practically one of a kind. The following clinical vignettes will serve to indicate the large variety of cases likely to be encountered in an outpatient setting.

An occasional patient may not feel free initially to say what is wanted, afraid that a particular request will be regarded as unacceptable because only certain symptoms are proper "tickets for admission." Such was true in the case described below.

> *A student nurse became rather vague when asked about her reasons for seeking treatment and merely mentioned some indecision about whether to marry or complete nurses' training first. Only after she inquired about her diagnosis and received an answer did the situation become clear. She then explained that her father had been diagnosed as having schizophrenia and her roommate had labelled her (the patient) a schizophrenic. Although she did not think the diagnosis fit her, because she had no delusions or hallucinations, she still wanted an expert's opinion. When informed that there was no evidence for the diagnosis of schizophrenia, she appeared greatly relieved, said that was all she wanted, thanked the psychiatrist, and left.*

The following instance is one in which psychotherapy was sought for an unusual reason.

> *A 42-year-old woman came to a psychiatric clinic seeking help in coping with feelings engendered by the imminent departure from the city of a man friend of 10 years. Their relationship, which had been sexual for the first few years,*

had developed into a close, platonic friendship. What made the situation so difficult, the patient explained, was that her friend was married and therefore she could not talk to others about her feelings. When asked what type of work her friend did, it was learned that he was a preacher in the church she attended. He had encouraged her to seek psychiatric help, recognizing that only in the confidential situation of psychotherapy, and nowhere else, would she be able to speak freely about her loss and deal with her grief.

In the following instance, the therapist could infer what the patient was seeking even though the patient herself was aware only of reaching out in the dark for a helping hand.

June came to the clinic following her fourth separation from John, her live-in friend of five years. As on previous occasions, John was trying to persuade her to return. He promised to reform in certain respects, and he also stated that he would seriously consider her wish to have children. She did not know what to do—to stay away or return.

It is noteworthy that this was the first time June had sought psychiatric help. At the time of the three previous separations she went through an internal struggle but in each instance gave in to John's entreaties and went back to live with him. And shortly after they resumed living together, he would break his promises.

The fact that this time June came to a psychiatrist immediately suggested that she might be looking for support so she could take a stand that she had not been able to take on her own. Possibly she hoped that the psychiatrist would bolster her resolve so that she could hold to her decision. Perhaps she wanted to be told: "Look, you have fallen back into the same pit three times. Don't you think it's time to 'split' for good?" There may be, of course, other reasons she sought psychiatric help, and it would be important to listen intently for clues that might point in a particular direction.

June stated she was inclined to consider John's latest promises because never before had he been willing to talk about having children. The fact that he was willing now, she thought, made the situation different. The story of "this time it is or will be different" is like the familiar plea of the alcoholic who, each time he swears off liquor, declares that this time it will be different—but it rarely is.

Therapy here might first consist of confirming June's decision to break off her relationship and then bolstering her resolve. Then, if she terminates her relationship with John, she could be offered a more definitive type of psychotherapy—therapy that would help her to understand why she had continued to return to a person like John and why she had remained with him for so long.

Psychiatric treatment may be sought to appease someone else. Although the "someone else" is most often a family member, it is sometimes a physician, as in the following case.

> *Ms. B, 53 years old and a widow, was referred to a psychiatric clinic by her internist who told her, as he had in the past, that her physical condition was good but that she needed psychiatric treatment for her nervous state. The "nervous state" consisted mainly of a long list of hypochondriacal complaints that dated back many years and that she tolerated with remarkable forbearance. In questioning Ms. B it soon became evident that she agreed to see a psychiatrist only to appease her physician to whom she had been most grateful over the years. She did not seek psychiatric treatment; all she wanted was a statement that would satisfy her internist and keep her in his good graces.*

At times seeking psychotherapy represents acting out behavior. For example, one woman, when angry at her husband, would schedule psychotherapy appointments. Over a period of time, it became clear that she regarded these appointments as a means of demonstrating to her husband that he had injured her and therefore she needed to seek treatment. In addition he was being "punished in that he had to pay the fees."

Are the Patient's Expectations Realistic?

To some extent probably all patients expect magical help and idyllic results from psychotherapy. There is a crucial difference, however, between expectations that are paramount and unchecked and those that show only at the edges and are counterbalanced by realistic objectives. In the latter case the unrealistic expectations can be recognized and dispelled during psychotherapy; in the former they may create a serious problem that is not easily resolved.

When patients expect psychotherapy to accomplish tasks for which it was not designed, they are obviously being unrealistic.

An example is the case of a 30-year-old man, Mr. K, who sought treatment because he was convinced that his wife would desist from having affairs if he were the perfect mate.

This man's outlook immediately suggested the following questions: Why did he blame himself and assume that the problem was his? Why did he not entertain the possibility that his wife had a problem or that they did not behave according to the same code of conduct? Clearly, his expectations seemed grossly unrealistic. It appeared that he was reaching for straws, and he was told so. He left stating he would think matters over before doing anything further. Three months later he called to report that he had decided to divorce his wife because she had flatly refused to remain faithful to him.

It could be argued that Mr. K's reaction—the assumption that his wife would be faithful to him if he were the perfect husband—is "neurotic" and that this kind of psychopathology should be treated. However, he did not seek help for that purpose, and it is unlikely that he would have accepted treatment in terms other than his own. Whatever the approach, the issue to be faced and dealt with was the unrealistic nature of Mr. K's expectations.

The Patient's Expectations of the Therapist-Patient Relationship

As described in Chapter 2, the patient realistically may be concerned about the therapist's training and competence. In addition to biographical information that is requested directly, more personal information may be sought indirectly. The following is an account of such an instance.

> *Ms. A, 24 years old and divorced, came to the clinic because of depression that began after she was jilted by a man. In spite of the fact that the depression lifted when she began seeing another man, she decided to continue with an evaluation for therapy because of her awareness that she repeatedly became involved with men who hurt her. She was personable and pretty, and she took evident care in her appearance.*
>
> *When Ms. A was asked if she had any questions, she stated that the other night on television she heard a man state that he had never seen a psychiatrist who did not need a psychiatrist. (It can be inferred that this statement refers to*

> *her therapist. Perhaps she was asking him, indirectly to be sure: How stable or emotionally healthy are you?)*
>
> *Ms. A then commented that when new merchandise came into the store where she worked, she was always thrilled because she liked what she did. She wondered, "Do psychiatrists look on a new patient as new merchandise?" (The patient wondered how her therapist viewed her. Was he "thrilled" to have someone new? But did he see her as merchandise?)*
>
> *When the therapist said that he did not understand Ms. A's question, she said, "What I mean is: How involved do you get with your patients? How warm are you? Or, do you stay cold?" (The patient obviously was wondering about what type of relationship they would have—how much involvement? How warm or how cold would he be?)*
>
> *At this point the therapist was aware of becoming defensive. He stated, "I get involved to an extent, but because I have to remain objective, I can't get too involved with my patients."*
>
> *The patient's next question was, "Have you been psychoanalyzed yourself?" Instead of answering, the therapist said that they would talk about this later. He felt as though he were backed against the wall.*

The comment about psychiatrists who need a psychiatrist and the question about a personal psychoanalysis fit together. Ms. A moved from a less specific to a more specific question. As a result the question could now be posed to her in personal terms: "You are wondering if I will be able to help you or if my own problems and needs will interfere."

It seems likely that Ms. A's earlier question about whether the therapist would see her like new merchandise related to her notion (previously expressed) that men were attracted to her body but were not interested in her as a person.

The nature of the relationship the patient seeks with the therapist may be discerned from the type of relationship sought in analogous situations. The following three instances are examples:

> *A young woman spoke of a teacher who expected his pupils to find out for themselves what had taken him 50 years to learn. That, she stated, was not her idea of education.*

A young man complained, "You know, my father is getting more distant. . . . I can't ask him for advice anymore because he always tells me to do what I think is best."

Another young man made clear the type of relationship he was seeking when he said, "Why won't he [his boss] explain things to me, go over things with me? He could do in 15 minutes what it takes me a half day to do. It's easier to be shown than to discover things on my own."

It is important that therapist and patient reach an agreement on the nature of the therapist-patient relationship. Problems will arise if the patient assumes that the relationship will be guidance-cooperation whereas the therapist assumes that it will be mutual participation (Szasz and Hollender 1956).

An even more serious problem will arise if the patient pretends to be a mutual participant in the interest of obtaining dependent gratification that comes with guidance-cooperation. This situation might be likened to that of the Marranos in Spain. At the time of the Inquisition many Jews seemingly converted to Catholicism but secretly continued to practice Judaism in their basements. Similarly, some patients pretend to be mutual participants to please or placate their therapists but actually seek guidance and dependent gratification.

In the following instance, a young woman was in conflict about the type of relationship she wanted, as often is the case.

At the end of Ms. R's first appointment, she asked for suggestions on how to handle some problems that were likely to arise before her next appointment. She had mentioned that, in her previous therapy, she was pleased when the therapist gave her "permission" to engage in sex and provided "direction" for coping with certain issues. She had also mentioned, however, that she did not want to be under her parents' thumb, that she was struggling to free herself and gain more autonomy. A step in this direction was taken when she supported herself financially while attending college the previous year.

These conflicting statements made it clear that the patient was pulled in two directions: one to find an indulgent parent who would tell her what to do and the other to find someone who would encourage her to emancipate herself. This conflict should be highlighted during the evaluation period. If the patient initially favors emancipation but later wants the therapist to be an indulgent parent, it can be pointed out to her that this struggle clearly is within herself (intrapsychic). It is to be anticipated that the nature of the patient's relationship with her therapist, reflecting as it does her simultaneous wish to remain a child and to become an adult, will be a central issue in therapy—and in life.

Assessment of Ego Strength

Ego strength is an important quality to assess in determining a person's capacity for psychotherapy. Particularly with insight-oriented psychotherapy, there needs to be some capacity to tolerate frustration, a discipline for the stick-to-itiveness required, and the willingness at times to look at the more unpleasant aspects of oneself. There is no direct way to quantify ego strength (no "egomanometer"), but its qualities can be inferred by considering various aspects of a person's life history. For example, what was the person's school achievement, not only in terms of the number of years but in academic accomplishments that correlated with innate skills and abilities?

For persons who were in the military service, how did they handle the authoritarian structure or the stresses imposed by an adverse environment? What was the capability for leadership? Did the person have difficulty with discipline and was he or she able to advance at the usual rate or was there delayed or accelerated promotion?

In regard to employment, questions may be asked as to the length of each job. Were the nature of the job and the pay commensurate with the person's abilities? Was there difficulty with employers and/or coworkers?

The legal record is of importance, too. Has the patient had difficulty with the police, been arrested, or been jailed? Is there a record of repetitive traffic offenses such as reckless driving or driving under the influence of alcohol?

A history regarding use of mind-altering chemicals is essential. Does the patient use alcohol or other drugs and, if so, under what circumstances? Is there a history of habituation, either currently or in the past? Does the individual typically turn to drinking when under stress?

The quality of a person's interpersonal relationships is also an important measure of ego strength. This particular issue is so important that it is discussed below in detail.

Assessment of Interpersonal Relationships

A careful assessment of the nature of the person's present and previous interpersonal relationships is possibly the most important part of the evaluation for psychotherapy. There are several reasons for this. First, many if not most problems that present to psychotherapists are directly or indirectly related to a person's interpersonal relationships. For example, a person may seek help because of discomfort related to conflicts with a spouse, or may present for treatment because of severe grief and depression precipitated by the death of a loved one. The second consideration is that psychotherapy is probably more efficacious in influencing changes in interpersonal relationships than in changing entrenched behavioral or characterological patterns. Although it is not a firm rule, many patients report, when therapy has been "successful," that the major change in their life is in the quality of their interpersonal relationships.

Finally, psychotherapy is built on an interpersonal relationship, and the course of psychotherapy will be determined to a large extent by the patient's prior interpersonal relationships. The fact that psychotherapy is built on an interpersonal relationship probably accounts for its effectiveness in problems of human relatedness. The therapeutic situation represents an "in vivo" laboratory setting in which one can both investigate and influence the patient's capacity to relate to others.

The therapist should evaluate the prospective patient's relationships with a variety of different persons in the past and in different situations to determine the presence of continuing patterns. The relationships with peers may reflect earlier relationships with siblings. How a person relates to authority figures should be examined, keeping in mind that the prototypes of these relationships were the relationships with parents. In addition, one should examine how the person relates to those persons who are perceived to be in a subordinate role and to determine patterns of relationships with those of the same sex as well as the opposite sex (Strupp and Binder 1986).

In surveying these relationships one should look for evidence of conflicts around certain themes. Among these themes are topics related to anger, aggressiveness, and assertiveness. For example, does the patient have difficulty controlling anger or, on the contrary, is anger being repressed? Is the patient able to express anger toward some persons and not toward others? Is there a pattern in this regard?

Another common area of conflict is that of passivity and dependence. Does the patient look toward other people to take care of him or her? Can the patient engage in an interdependent relationship with another person and enjoy intimacy and emotional warmth? Again, is there a pattern in this regard? For example, does a patient exhibit passivity and dependence with women but not with men? Is the patient able to express affectionate emotions, tender loving feelings, and yearnings? Is there the capacity for playfulness and spontaneity? How are sexual impulses and feelings handled? Is there a capacity for pleasure and enjoyment versus constriction of impulses and feelings?

Not all of the topics mentioned for assessing interpersonal relationships can be or need be explored during the evaluation period. Some priority might be assigned. For instance, it is likely to be more important at this stage to learn about the relationship with a previous therapist than to hear about how sexual impulses and feelings are handled.

Coping Mechanisms

People employ different ways of coping with the stress in their lives. It is the pattern of these coping mechanisms that, to a large extent, determines our definitions and descriptions of character. Defense mechanisms tend to be quite stable over time and may predict the capability of a person to adapt to life, to handle stressors, and to maintain self-esteem (Vaillant et al. 1986). Identifying these mechanisms is an important part of assessing the capability for particular types of psychotherapy and how the therapy is structured. For example, patients who are prone to act out when under stress tend to be less suitable for reconstructive therapies, which often elicit anxiety during the therapeutic work.

Reaction to Losses

Separation and losses are very important in determining emotional responses and the quality of relationships with other persons. For example, is a person fearful of becoming intimately involved with another person because of repeated losses and painful separations in the past? One should look carefully for evidence of losses or conflicts in childhood, such as the death of a parent or other significant person, parental divorce, frequent moves, birth of a sibling(s), and starting school. In regard to starting school, two major events stand out as being especially prone to conflict. The first is starting school for the very first time (kindergarten or first grade) and the second is leaving home for college. Losses during adolescence, which are often inappropriately minimized, should be investigated. For example, these include disappointments in academic, athletic, and social competition as well as in initial romantic ventures. Losses in adulthood are also important, such as deaths of parents and/or siblings, the patient's own separations or divorces, the death of a spouse, and major career changes.

Relationships with Prior Psychotherapists

Many patients have previously been in psychotherapy with another therapist. It is important that the quality of that interaction be explored during the evaluation period. Was it regarded as a positive or negative experience? Questions to be asked are: What did the patient learn from the experience? How is he or she different as a result of psychotherapy? What type of behavior was expected during psychotherapy? This last question is very important because it often sets the tone or the expectations of the prospective patient with the new therapist. At times a prior experience may have been extremely traumatic, for example, if there was a sexual encounter with the therapist or if the therapist died during the course of psychotherapy.

The following case note is one in which there was not only a change in therapists but also a change in the therapist-patient relationship—from guidance-cooperation to mutual participation.

> *A patient said to her new therapist, "You open the door for me; he [her previous therapist] would carry me through." During the previous week a change had come over the patient, a change she did not understand and found difficult to put into words. Somehow she felt that the therapist had gotten through to her. This past week her mood was much more even than usual. Although she did not like it when her husband took a nap every evening, she did not let it upset her and affect everything else. In speaking of her work as a kindergarten teacher, recently she had done less instructing and provided more opportunities for self-expression by her pupils; this method appealed to her. At first she despaired that some children would ever produce, but she was*

surprised and gratified when after a time they did—and they did so beautifully.

The therapist suggested that the difference this week indicated that she was more aware of her own internal resources and consequently had less need to lean on her husband who previously had to be God-like and on duty all the time. She commented that she thought that she finally understood her therapist's method. He works with her like she works with her pupils. Her first therapist had reassured her and built her up directly. Perhaps that was what she needed then. Now she has been made to realize she has some strengths within herself.

Relationship with the Therapist During the Evaluation

The patient's behavior toward the therapist during the evaluation period may be highly informative about how the patient relates with others and in predicting future behavior. For example, did the patient make an effort to be controlling in the relationship? Was there evasiveness? Was there a passive expectation of help? Was advice requested? Was there seductiveness in dress or manner? Was the prospective patient introspective or pensive? If there was more than one session for the evaluation, was there a change from session to session? Did the patient bring in new material based on a thoughtful reevaluation of what was discussed at the prior session?

Trial Interpretations

During the course of the evaluation, the therapist may attempt to connect some historical issues for the prospective patient. At times there may be some confrontations or interpretations of the material presented. As mentioned before, these might be regarded as "trial balloons," and the therapist must closely observe the patient's response to this material. Was the response an immediate denial? Did the patient provide important additional information, or did the trial interpretation evoke defensiveness?

The Developmental History

For the purpose of an assessment, some therapists recommend obtaining a chronological history, beginning as far back in the past as possible and moving forward, from one developmental stage to the next, to the present. In our opinion, such an approach hardly seems necessary and is not likely to be productive.

The problem in prediction based solely on a developmental history is highlighted by the following account: A mother wrote to her 18-year-old son, "Oh, ——, what a harum scarum fellow you are! You really must give up being so childish." She also described him as a "lazy-boy—and such a foolish one!" She added, "I don't see how he is to pass his exam if he goes on like this." His father chided him for forgetting to write "Dear Father" instead of "Dear Papa," and angrily harangued him for his bad English as well as for hinting for a bigger allowance (Leslie 1969).

This young man's future hardly seemed promising. He was regarded as immature for his years, less than a diligent scholar, and not even skilled in the use of his native tongue. What might mental health workers have predicted for him besides mediocrity, unhappiness, and disappointment—perhaps depression, marital difficulties, emotional problems, or worse? Certainly few would have predicted a successful future, and no one in his right mind would have guessed that he, Winston Churchill, would become the greatest British leader of the twentieth century.

If the focus in history-taking is maintained on the here-and-now, blueprints drawn in the past that play a substantial part in shaping the present can be discerned. It is not the past itself that is of concern but only the part that obtrudes and creates problems in the present.

The Formulation

As mentioned at the beginning of this chapter, a psychiatric diagnosis is necessary but not sufficient in evaluating a patient for psychotherapy. In addition there is a need for an assessment that takes into account how the presenting symptoms relate to the patient's entire life course, character structure, coping styles, and relationships with others. If possible, the formulation should be framed in terms of patterns of interpersonal relatedness. If the therapist clearly understands the issues, it should then be possible to construct a brief summary which can be provided for the patient in his or her own language. For example, a man seeking therapy for the symptom of intermittent anxiety might be provided with the following formulation: "Your symptom of anxiety appears to come on when you get angry at your boss. It seems that you are afraid that your anger will break out. We know that as a child you were severely punished if you became angry at your parents. The two circumstances certainly sound like they are related."

This above formulation is obviously somewhat simplistic; patients will have more than one issue that is important. However, it is essential in explaining the formulation to the patient that it be presented in a clear manner and that it have immediate meaning. The use of jargon should be avoided.

A formulation must take into account certain features outside the psychodynamic determinants of the patient's life, for example, biological predispositions and life circumstances beyond the patient's control. The psychodynamic formulation can be framed from more than one theoretical position (e.g., an object relations versus a self psychology model). It should serve to provide guidelines for the treatment and anticipate the unfolding of certain behaviors in the therapeutic process (Perry et al. 1987).

Selecting the Appropriate Approach

If a therapist becomes wedded to one type of treatment there is the danger that the patient will be expected to fit the treatment rather than the treatment fit the patient. Then, instead of an evaluation to select the appropriate approach, a trial period serves to determine if the "treatment of choice" can be used. For example there are clinicians today who recommend a trial period of brief psychotherapy for every patient regarded as suitable for psychotherapy. This approach is similar to that taken by Freud (1913), who recommended in selecting analysands that the verbal material produced during a period of a week or two be used for "taking a sounding."

In selecting the appropriate type of treatment the following questions should be addressed:

1. Is the patient seeking help with an acute problem or distress, or does the patient wish to make personality changes? The former might be amenable to brief therapy and the latter to long-term therapy.

2. Is the patient capable of facing unconscious forces that might be revealed with an uncovering technique, or is the patient better served by an approach that covers over and supports?
3. Is the patient oriented to dealing with personal problems, or is the patient intent on resolving marital conflicts? In the former instance there is a willingness to let the marital chips fall where they may; in the latter the goal is to resolve differences or to decide on a divorce.
4. Is the patient willing to scrutinize problem areas, or is the patient only willing to take medications? Many patients, of course, are willing to do both.

Often several factors in combination suggest that a particular approach is indicated. For example, brief psychotherapy might be chosen if the onset of a problem is sudden, the previous adjustment and ability to relate are good, the difficulty seems relatively circumscribed, and the motivation for working in psychotherapy is strong. Not all circumscribed disorders, however, are equally responsive. For instance monosymptomatic hypochondriacal psychosis is especially resistant to psychotherapy.

The following generalization can be made: States resulting from loss or fear may be helped by supportive, cathartic, and interpretative forms of psychotherapy, whereas paranoid states involving grossly distorted notions held with great conviction may be resistant to all nonmedicinal interventions.

As has been emphasized, personal motivation may be of overriding significance. Therapists should be on the lookout for patients who appear to be highly motivated but lack tenacity. They are the ones who approach new projects with great enthusiasm and dramatic intensity but in a short while lose interest, disengage, and turn to another pursuit. This recurrent pattern, aptly described as being like a *brushfire*, is almost certain to appear in therapy. If forewarned, some of these patients may make an effort to discover the determinants of the pattern instead of disengaging and turning to another pursuit.

A second pattern for which therapists should be on the lookout is a *readiness to relinquish control* and to assume that the psychotherapeutic process will bring about a desired state. An example is the obese patient who believes that it will no longer be necessary to diet because psychotherapy will take care of the situation. This incorrect assumption and misplaced faith should be pointed out.

In a third pattern the patient quickly develops a *clinging relationship* to a therapist. Safirstein (1972), in describing this pattern, stated, "The clinging patient uses the relationship with the doctor as the vehicle in which to express his need to be attached and, once ensconced in this relationship, he cannot be moved." At the outset he appears to be a "good" patient. He flatters the therapist's professional vanity by reporting marked improvement. He seldom complains, he pays his bill on time if he is a private patient, and if he is a clinic patient he may praise his therapist to other patients in the waiting room. What appears to be a patient "moving in therapy" turns out to be one extremely difficult to disengage because he falls back on disturbing somatic symptoms, helplessness, or suicidal threats. This pattern should be identified in the patient's history. In particular, a paucity of relationships and involvements that are intense and have a clinging quality are warnings that should be heeded. Outside relationships should be encouraged, and the extent of the therapist-patient involvement should be carefully monitored from the very beginning.

In a fourth pattern, patients whose lives are dull and unfulfilling are prone to make therapy a *way of life* instead of an aid to living. They invest their energy and seek their fulfillment in the therapy hours and react to the time in between as a waiting period or a hiatus. A history of previous overinvestment in treatment is a warning that should be heeded.

In a fifth pattern, referred to as *fool's mate*, a male therapist is "taken in" by or opens himself up to a female patient who is young, attractive, intelligent, articulate, and personable. In spite of what appeared to be a promising beginning, little progress is made. The patient goes through motions in the interest of obtaining supplies such as special attention or dependent gratification.

Summary

Before determining whether to proceed with psychotherapy and, if so, what type, the patient must be carefully evaluated. The therapist should go beyond a DSM-III-R diagnosis to estimate the patient's ability to work in treatment. This includes an assessment of the patient's ego strength, coping mechanisms, interpersonal relationships, and initial responses to the therapist. The patient's expectations of desired results from therapy and of the process must be determined. A psychodynamic formulation, derived from the evaluation, serves to provide the guidelines for the therapeutic plan. There are certain patterns of patient behavior that on the surface initially appear to be motivation for change but, in reality, portend difficulty over the course of a psychotherapy.

4

Agreement: The Therapeutic Contract

Patients with varying degrees of acute distress present themselves asking for help. The greater the emergency the less distinct will be the divisions labelled "evaluation," "agreement," and "beginning of treatment." In critical situations there is little the therapist can do other than to indicate a willingness to be helpful and to take steps to cope with the pressing issues of the moment. The latter may be accomplished by talking, administering medication, or arranging for hospitalization.

In less acute situations, following a period reserved for diagnosis, evaluation, and treatment planning—usually one to three appointments—the therapist should be in a position to make a recommendation on how to proceed. If the recommendation is for psychotherapy, the type should be named: psychoanalysis; insight-oriented, brief, focal, or supportive psychotherapy; marital or group therapy; or a combination of medication and psychotherapy, to list only some of the options.

The Procedure

To draw a vivid picture of the nature of psychotherapy with words is a difficult task. The roles of the patient and the therapist need to be sketched with attention paid to what is expected of the therapist as well as what is expected of the patient. No longer is it acceptable, if it ever was, for the therapist to sit like a sphinx, attentive but silent and impassive, as the patient talks on and on. It is still possible, however, that the therapist will offer too little and the patient will expect too much.

The objective of treatment—symptom relief, resolution of pressing problems, or characterological change—should be described. Like other treatment procedures, the proposal of psychotherapy should be presented in a manner in keeping with the guidelines for informed consent. (We are considering only those patients who are capable of participating in decision making.)

A realistic assessment of possible benefits should be made and communicated to the patient. Much like patients who request a rhinoplasty believing that their lives will be remarkably changed by a "new" nose, some patients will request psychotherapy believing that their "new" personality will have a dramatic effect on their relationships with others. Patients should be told what they can expect if psychotherapy is undertaken and what they can expect if it is not undertaken. For some patients, treatment might be helpful but far from mandatory. Accordingly, they should be informed that for them psychotherapy is an elective procedure. Finally, the risks should be mentioned. For example, the patient may make changes that disrupt the central relationship in a marriage. Not all reactions to psychotherapy are positive, and the possibility of an adverse outcome should be considered.

The type of psychotherapy recommended and the goal to be reached determine the particular procedure to be followed.

Insight-Oriented Psychotherapy

For the patient treated with insight-oriented psychotherapy, the primary objective will be increased self-knowledge. In keeping with this orientation, the prospective patient will be informed that the focus will be on understanding how old patterns or "blueprints" influence or shape present-day living and on discovering the sources of persistent feelings of anxiety, guilt, shame, and depression. Because of the desirability of personalizing the presentation, the therapist should refer to problems that were mentioned by the patient.

In insight-oriented psychotherapy the prospective patient is told that he or she will be encouraged to speak of whatever comes to his or her mind, with as little selecting and editing as possible. The therapist, in turn, as a trained participant-observer, will strive to add a dimension to the patient's productions. Like a decoder, the therapist will attempt to unravel the unconscious meaning of the messages and convey the information to the patient for consideration.

Patients who have heard about free association may inquire about it. Freud (1909), in discussing free association, stated, "I made him [the patient] pledge himself to submit to the one and only condition of the treatment—namely, to say everything that came into his head, even if it was *unpleasant* to him, or seemed *unimportant* or *irrelevant* or *senseless*." (See Chapter 6.)

Although Freud stated that there was one and only one condition of treatment, other psychoanalysts promulgated additional rules. One of the best known is the injunction against patients making major changes in their lives while in treatment, including marriage, divorce, opening a new business, or changing career direction. The concern that gave rise to this rule was that patients might plunge headlong in a particular direction as the result of feelings stimulated by treatment at a time when regression had impaired their judgment.

The imposition of the rule that patients were not to make major decisions was no doubt introduced to protect them. But patients require protection only if they are encouraged to regress and become infantilized. The danger of precipitous action based on feelings of the moment exists for persons who are not in psychotherapy as well as those who are. At least patients have the opportunity to discuss their plans and to consider how the proposed change will influence their lives. Further, it should be explained to patients that because of the nature of the goals and the techniques employed to reach those goals, they will be expected to take the initiative in therapy and should not expect the therapist to provide advice or instructions as to which topics to discuss. Finally, there should be some estimate of the time required to reach the goals desired. No firm promise can be made, but it would be deceptive to imply that therapy might be completed in months when experience indicates years are necessary for the resolution of some problems.

Focal Psychotherapy

When patients seek help in coping with specific problems that should be amenable to psychotherapy, they should be informed that the focus on the specific problem will be maintained, the extent of the area scrutinized will be limited, and the area to be worked on will be defined as distinctly as possible. In this respect the therapist is likely to be more directive in defining subject matter than in insight-oriented psychotherapy. It is likely that with focal therapy there will be an admixture of techniques utilized for insight-oriented psychotherapy and supportive psychotherapy (see below). As a general rule the time limits of focal therapy are stated much more specifically than for other forms of psychotherapy. These may be either in terms of time (e.g., three months) or the number of sessions (e.g., 12 sessions). Such a limit helps to maintain the therapeutic focus.

Supportive Psychotherapy

With supportive psychotherapy the therapist attempts to help patients utilize their customary coping mechanisms as much as possible. With this therapeutic approach the focus is not on the unconscious determinants of behavior, but rather on coping with day-to-day stresses. Patients for whom supportive psychotherapy is proposed should be told in general and nontechnical terms what to expect. For example, a woman whose husband recently left her and threatened her with divorce might be told that during this difficult transition period in her life it would be helpful for her to have an objective listener with whom she could ventilate feelings (catharsis) and discuss decisions that must be made (problem solving). Another example would be a man who, while struggling with angry feelings toward an employer, has associated tension headaches. A proposed treatment plan might include helping the patient with stress management (learning techniques of relaxation or sublimation) and understanding more effective ways of managing anger (assertiveness training).

The possibilities are many but the point is that therapy should have a direction, and patients should understand what is being proposed as a treatment plan. With supportive psychotherapy the length of treatment can be brief and at times it is therapeutic to limit it (e.g., with a patient in whom dependency and regression might be encouraged by prolonged treatment). It is not unusual, however, to see patients in supportive psychotherapy off and on, for months or years, depending on the amount of stress in their lives.

Management

By management we mean a strategy or a course of action based on an understanding of the patient's psychodynamics. It should be differentiated from the casual prescription of advice (i.e., take a vacation). Taken into account is an understanding of what is likely to be the unconscious meaning of a nonmedicinal prescription. (For examples of the use of management, see Chapter 12.) The response to management will determine if a more definitive type of treatment should be prescribed. If such seems in order, the original therapeutic agreement should be renegotiated.

Practical Arrangements

Payment

When questions have been answered and the patient accepts, tentatively at least, the therapist's proposal for treatment, it is time to deal with practical matters. The fee for each session may have been stated in response to an inquiry before the first appointment or mentioned at the end of the first session. If it has not been, it should be stated now. A private practitioner may have a fixed fee, whereas a clinic is likely to have a sliding scale based on income, family size, and perhaps other factors. Bills are usually sent at the end of each month and, as is customary in most communities, payment is expected by the fifteenth of the month. Fees for psychotherapy should, in general, be handled in a manner consistent with the local customs in regard to medical services. At times this will include payment at each visit, particularly in large clinics. Such a routine may place too much emphasis on monetary considerations, however, and hence be objectionable in some settings.

It has sometimes been stated that if the patient is to derive appreciable benefit from psychotherapy, he or she must pay a fee and ideally one that pinches slightly. Such a condition, it is argued, ensures or fortifies motivation. If it is important for therapists to work on a fee-for-service basis, it probably is not for the reason just mentioned. In our society monetary payment is essential if the patient is not to feel beholden for a gift or charity. If services are not recompensed monetarily, patients may feel compelled to "pay" in some other way, for example, by being the good child or outstanding pupil. Payment in this form may be more costly than money because of its effect on self-expression and the freedom to pursue personal goals in therapy.

This is not to say that it is essential for patients to pay directly for services. Patients in a clinic may pay a low fee or no fee without incurring a feeling of obligation because the therapist is compensated financially by a governmental or private agency. Similarly, patients may pay for their sessions, partly or entirely, through insurance coverage without incurring a personal sense of indebtedness.

Schedule

The length of each session (often referred to as an "hour") is usually 45 or 50 minutes but may be 15 or 30 minutes. The length of the session should be mentioned in detailing the practical arrangements. So too should the number of visits, which may vary roughly from five times a week to once a month.

It is desirable to establish a regular schedule so that both parties can plan ahead. From time to time, of course, changes may be made to accommodate the needs of therapist or patient. If the therapist takes a vacation at the same time each year, this should be mentioned. And if the therapist knows that he or she will be completing training and moving away within one year, this should also be mentioned.

Some therapists charge patients in insight-oriented psychotherapy for missed appointments if the patient's vacation time does not coincide with theirs. Such a policy is clearly unfair when a patient either must forego an out-of-town vacation or pay for missed hours if the vacation dates acceptable to the patient's employer do not coincide with the therapist's vacation time. In this situation, the therapist may be unwilling to recognize the possibility that a one-sided stand is responsible for the patient's justifiable anger and is not a matter for analysis. The matter of vacation time should be discussed and ground rules set as part of the agreement.

Missed Appointments

Closely related to vacation time are canceled or missed appointments. Freud (1913) stated, "In regard to time, I adhere strictly to the principle of leasing a definite hour. Each patient is allotted a particular hour of my working day; it belongs to him and he is liable for it, even if he does not make use of it." Some therapists today contend, as Freud did, that regular hours are reserved for the patient and these hours must be paid for whether they are used or not. No exceptions are made for illnesses, deaths in the family, or babysitter problems. Thus, there can be no legitimate absence—at least for the patient.

If the therapist were willing to grant that some absences are legitimate, how will it be determined which ones are warranted and which are unwarranted? Occasionally it might be very difficult. But must the determination of whether the absence is warranted be precise? If the patient states that an absence was due to forgetting or oversleeping, such an absence would be regarded as unwarranted and payment for the time would be expected. If the patient was unable to find a babysitter but acknowledges that she made little effort to locate one, she would be charged for the missed hour.

Missed appointments or chronic tardiness may become a major issue during the process of therapy, and it is therefore essential that policies in this regard be determined at the beginning of therapy. The issues raised by this behavior and techniques to deal with them are detailed in Chapter 14.

Converting the Patient

In the process of reaching an agreement it is necessary to ascertain what the patient hopes to achieve and what he or she is willing to do to achieve it. If the objective is symptom relief, must the approach be a direct one (the use of a behavior modification technique to treat a phobia, for example) or can it be indirect (the use of dynamic psychotherapy to bring about a characterological change that may secondarily affect the symptom)?

The nature of the therapist-patient relationship that is being sought must also be taken into consideration (Szasz and Hollender 1956). Does the patient want to be told what to do (guidance-co-operation), or does the patient want to be helped to help himself or herself (mutual participation)?

Fundamental to arriving at an agreement is the patient's orientation. Seldom is it possible to convert a patient successfully from one approach to another. Therefore, it is necessary to understand what the patient's expectations are.

In the following instance, a patient and her therapist had very different expectations.

> *A 28-year-old woman, when asked what she sought in therapy, said, "Relief from depressions." The depressions came on only when she lost a job or a man left her, and they lasted no longer than a few days. At the time she called for an appointment in a psychiatric clinic, she had just lost a job, and for the first time she had been unable to find another job immediately. Based on the patient's account, the therapist saw her as having what has sometimes been called a "fate neurosis," a disorder in which outside forces are held responsible for events that happen to the patient. The events in this case included repeatedly losing jobs, two out-of-wedlock children by two different men, and drifting from one masochistic relationship to another. The patient stated that she sought treatment to obtain relief from a symptom, but the therapist's focus was elsewhere. Impressed by her characterological pattern, he thought in terms of altering the*

patient's picture of herself, as a leaf in the breeze with little ability to determine where she might go and what she might do.

Clearly, the patient and the therapist did not agree on the treatment objective. If this disparity went unnoticed, there would be the danger of working at cross purposes and accomplishing very little.

All too often when it is assumed that a patient has been converted from one approach to another, the result is like that described in the following clinical vignette.

A young man sought help to obtain relief from some symptoms so that he would be able to fly again. His therapist tried to convert him into an analytic patient. After several months the patient stopped paying his bill. Finally the therapist presented an ultimatum: pay by a set date or treatment would stop. At the final hour the patient complained about an auto mechanic who overhauled his car and charged a large sum but did not fix the part of the car that was of concern to the patient. The message was clear.

Changing the Original Agreement

When the original agreement has been fulfilled but a desire to continue is expressed by the patient or recommended by the therapist, how should they proceed? In most instances a new agreement involving both the goal and the nature of the relationship should be negotiated or transfer to another therapist should be arranged. If the nature of the relationship is to be changed, as for example, from guidance-cooperation to mutual participation, a transfer to another therapist is generally advisable. As long as the patient remains with the original therapist, much time and energy is likely to be expended in an effort to perpetuate the old relationship.

In the following instance, therapy was continued without renegotiating the contract after the terms of the original agreement had been met.

Mrs. D came to the door of Dr. K's apartment one evening and asked to come in so she could talk to him. Mrs. D, attractive and personable, had been in treatment for three months. The goal had been to see her for six weekly appointments to help her cope with some pressing family problems and to find relief from her dysphoric mood. When the original objectives had been achieved, Mrs. D expressed a desire to continue in therapy to learn more about herself, and Dr. K acquiesced. Over time she telephoned him more and more often to ask for advice and support. Also, her request for more frequent appointments was granted and she was then seen twice a week.

At the door to Dr. K's apartment, Mrs. D appeared upset as she entreated him to let her come in. What should he do? Here was a situation for which he was not prepared. On the spot, he decided that he could not—indeed, should not—permit the patient to come in. To let her down gently he said that she could see the resident-on-call in the emergency room, or he could arrange to see her there later. She heard the message clearly, was not at all pleased, and left in a huff.

At Mrs. D's next appointment, the recent encounter at Dr. K's apartment was discussed. She spoke of her great affection for him, commenting that he was warmer and more understanding than her husband.

In this instance the relationship had been permitted to grow too intensely personal, and as a consequence the psychotherapy had threatened to become nontherapeutic or even destructive. Dr. K, by drawing the line and making it clear that he would not give in to Mrs. D's entreaty, acted appropriately.

In Mrs. D's case, not only had therapy continued without a new agreement after the short-term goal had been reached, but the patient had been permitted (perhaps even encouraged) to regress. The many phone calls for advice and support and the more frequent appointments resulted in an intensification of the dependency. After the episode at the apartment, Dr. K discussed the frequency of phone calls and appointments, and an understanding was reached. (Clearly, too, interpretation of the "transference" was in order—see Chapter 5.)

Psychiatric Evaluation

When a patient is sent for a psychiatric evaluation by an agency or person requesting a report, an understanding prior to the evaluation rather than a therapeutic agreement afterward is essential. The crucial issue is: Whose agent will the psychiatrist be?

Is he or she the agent of the patient or of the agency or person referring the patient?

If the psychiatrist agrees to do an evaluation and to render a report, he or she is the agent of the referring source, and this fact must be made absolutely clear to the patient at the very outset. In effect, a statement similar to the following should be made: "I have been asked by your employers to perform a psychiatric evaluation and to report my findings to them. You should understand that I am working for them and not for you. If I conclude that you might benefit from psychotherapy I will recommend it, but I will not be the one to treat you."

An evaluation is likely to be requested when students do not seem to be functioning up to their potential or when valued workers in a business are not as productive as they had been. Information may also be sought by draft boards, school admission committees, insurance companies, and lawyers.

In our society it is customary for those who engage or hire the services of a professional to pay for such services. Also, it is usually advisable to inform both parties that the written report may be shown to both of them. In this situation discretion should be exercised, but the patient cannot be ensured confidentiality.

Confidentiality

A few patients inquire about confidentiality, but most do not. Some patients either do not care or assume that they can rely on the discretion of their therapist. Whatever the therapists' stand and the patients' attitude, the subject usually should be brought up and discussed during the agreement phase. Both parties should understand the ground rules and be prepared to accept them. As mentioned in the previous section, if an evaluation is done for a third party, confidentiality is abrogated.

In cases in which patients are not capable of independent functioning, some information may have to be shared with family members who not only provide home care but also surveillance and supervision.

Only in insight-oriented psychotherapy, a private two-person encounter, is absolute confidentiality feasible and desirable. Therapists who wish to foster such a condition should be familiar with the laws pertaining to confidentiality in the state in which they practice. In some states there is considerable legal protection, in others very little. Little protection is typically provided in states in which psychiatrists are covered by the law applying broadly to physicians, with no separate statute applying specifically to psychiatric care. Therapists who are determined to maintain absolute confidentiality regardless of the law should ascertain what the consequences of their stand might be and decide if they are prepared to accept them.

If therapists state that they will be unwilling either to convey information or express a judgment to others, patients are likely to respond favorably, indicating that this is what they would prefer. Therapists should point out that perhaps the patients are thinking only of situations in which they would favor secrecy, not of those in which they would benefit from a letter written by the therapist to the dean of a college, an employer, or the secretary of a draft board requesting some special consideration.

It might be argued that therapists should be willing to write a very circumspect note, for instance, to the secretary of a draft board. The note might read, "Mr. J. Jones, who is in psychotherapy with me now, began his treatment eight months ago." On the surface such a statement seems innocuous, but is it? It is not if the members of the draft board or their medical advisers conclude that if Mr. Jones is in psychiatric treatment he must suffer from a psychiatric disorder that would disqualify him for induction into military service. This conclusion may or may not be correct. The significant issue is that deferment instead of increased self-knowledge may become the primary goal of psychotherapy and, as a consequence, the patient might only go through the motions of working on personal problems. There is no active draft program at present in the United States, but we cite this example to illustrate that therapists must always consider the patient's possible motives.

The Adolescent Patient's Parents

Before beginning psychotherapy with an adolescent patient—often a college student—it is important to meet with the parents if they are going to assume responsibility for the payment of the bills. Before arranging such a meeting, the therapist should assure the patient that nothing confidential will be disclosed. Whenever feasible the patient should be present at the meeting with the parents; when not feasible, he or she should be fully informed about what transpired. The parents should be told something about the type of treatment recommended, how it will be conducted, and the cost. Any question asked by the parents should be answered, provided that the patient's confidentiality is not abridged.

The parents are likely to find it reassuring to see and talk to the person with whom their son or daughter will be in treatment and to have some idea about the nature and objectives of the treatment. At the same time that they gain a picture of what they can expect, they also are made aware of what is expected of them.

Implicit Rules

A number of rules pertaining to psychotherapy are left unspoken. They can remain implicit because they are woven so firmly into the fabric of our culture that it would be belaboring the obvious to call attention to them. Patients know without being told that they will not be permitted to destroy office furnishings, disrobe, bring weapons to the therapist's office, or physically injure the therapist. To speak of such wishes or fantasies is permissible because patients are informed that they may speak of whatever comes to mind.

It is implicit that, if there is a palpable danger of harm to the therapist, the patient, or another person, the therapist has a responsibility to intervene. In doing so the therapist-patient relationship may be irreversibly altered. Emergency situations do require drastic measures, sometimes with unfortunate consequences. Such situations arise infrequently, yet the therapist must be prepared to act quickly and decisively.

Summary

With the initiation of psychotherapy there must be agreement between the patient and therapist as to the goals and the therapeutic process. This agreement is often called the "therapeutic contract." As part of this contract there should be a clear understanding of such matters as the scheduling of appointments, the payment of fees, and the limits of confidentiality. It is also important that the therapist understand whose agent he or she is and make certain the patient also understands.

5

Insight-Oriented Psychotherapy: Initiating Therapy and the Relationship

Insight-oriented psychotherapy can begin once an evaluation has been completed and an agreement on how to proceed has been reached.

Initiating the Therapeutic Relationship

During the pretherapy phase the patient may raise questions about the therapist *as a professional* (see Chapter 3), whereas in the beginning phase of therapy the patient usually tries to learn how to relate to the therapist *as a person.* In doing so the patient's approach is likely to be less direct than it was in obtaining information about professional competence. Moreover, it is likely to be studded with assumptions stemming from earlier experiences with father or mother figures.

It is extremely important for the therapist to look for indirect communications, oblique references, and analogies that suggest or make it clear how he or she is perceived. The patient's built-in assumptions should be pointed out. Failure to point them out may result in an interference with communication. This is particularly likely if the therapist is pictured as impatient, unsympathetic, or critical.

In terms of human relationships, psychotherapy presents a unique situation. One of its novel features is the explicit understanding that the patient will reveal a great deal about himself or herself and the therapist will reveal very little. In business encounters, after an exchange of social amenities, the conversation may move onto the shared ground of "shop talk." In social situations, two strangers brought together may chat about the weather, a news topic of the day, or mutual friends. Each soon recognizes what can be expected from the other. If they find common interests, they continue to converse; if not, they drift apart. But psychotherapy is different. No well-traveled and familiar path is available. Consequently, the patient may grope while looking for a path to follow.

Some patients ask how they should proceed. Others request that the therapist pose questions as a starter. Still others assume that they know what is expected of them. For example, a young woman, remembering what she had read and seen on television, launched into a detailed exposition of early memories and traumatic childhood experiences. Another woman, acting on her impression that sex is the root of all problems and the primary focus of therapists, recounted several sexual experiences in considerable detail (Hollender 1965).

The early stage of therapy may serve as a time for testing. As one way of testing, a patient may disclose "horrendous secrets." For example, one woman, after prefacing her remarks by stating that she had some terrible things to relate, said that she stole money as a schoolgirl, shoplifted (and was apprehended) as a young married woman, sometimes picked feces from her rectum with her fingers, and cheated once on an examination. Her explanation for why she blurted out all this was that she wanted to make certain that the therapist would not become disgusted with her later and "toss her out" of therapy. If he was not shocked by her awful disclosures, "his stomach probably would be strong enough" to tolerate her. She obviously regarded rejection while still only slightly involved as preferable to rejection after greater involvement.

Initial Expectations and Concerns

Patients often have unrealistic expectations when they enter psychotherapy. Only if these expectations are extreme or are held with great tenacity, however, do they become a serious impediment. As in popular soap operas, the patient sometimes has the notion that "life can be beautiful," and as in fairy tales, that one can "live happily ever after." Patients must first become aware of the nature and extent of their expectations and then strive to recalibrate or revise them.

Along with unrealistic expectations, at the outset of psychotherapy there are likely to be unrealistic concerns or fears. Some patients are afraid that it will be discovered that they are "crazy," others that they will appear ludicrous and evoke mirthful but secret laughter, and still others that a "monster"—something violent and evil—will emerge. These fears or concerns should be brought into the open, scrutinized, and, if possible, dispelled.

Reaction to the Procedure

During the early phase of psychotherapy, the reaction to the procedure itself may become significant. Patients who are told to speak of whatever they wish or to free associate (see Chapter 6) may feel the same type of uneasiness experienced by surgical patients before undergoing anesthesia. They think, "What will I blurt out or reveal about myself when my guard is down?"

During the early phase of psychotherapy, the patient may struggle with the question: What is therapy going to be like? If the question is only hinted at or alluded to, the therapist's task is to make it explicit. The following instance is illustrative.

> *A young man contrasted his experience in reading technical essays and light novels. With the former he struggled, reading them a little at a time; the latter he read in one pleasant sitting. In the context in which the patient made this statement, it could be surmised that he was asking: "What will psychotherapy be like? Will it be slow, laborious, and technical or easy to master, pleasant, and exciting?" By making this connection explicit, the therapist opened the subject for discussion.*

The Patient's Perceptions of the Therapist

The majority of patients neither ask for directions nor assume they know how to relate to the therapist. In striving to discern what the therapist is *really* like, they proceed to imagine what he is *possibly* like. This step—an important step—may be taken automatically and unconsciously. These patients, like a writer of fiction delineating characters, draw on their previous personal experiences.

It would be a mistake, however, to assume that the patients' characterizations are purely figments of their imagination. They no doubt correctly observe or discern some traits in their therapist and respond to them. Lewin (1965) stated, "Although the patient may obtain certain information from . . . publications or from gossip, his most convenient sources are the *nonverbal* clues afforded by the therapist and his office." Among the clues are the location of the therapist's office, the way it is furnished, and the magazines in the waiting room.

Although the therapist-patient relationship is interactive, for discussion purposes, encounters will be described first in which the patients' responses to their therapists are predominantly the products of their own preconceptions. Later instances will be described in which the patients' responses are to a substantial degree, or even largely, determined by their therapists' behavior and personality.

The following excerpt from an hour in the beginning phase of psychotherapy illustrates a young woman's effort to imagine what her therapist is like and then to cope with the straw man she has created.

> *Ms. B opened the hour by stating she knew why she did some of the things she did and then proceeded to describe and analyze them. Following this, she spoke of a clergyman who in counseling women sought to have them express their feelings to him instead of to their husbands. She observed that the person who does not have his own house in order points out other persons' faults. Such a person, she asserted, also tends to be pious and self-righteous.*

Ms. B did not directly state that she imagined that the therapist would be like the clergyman. In fact, she probably was not even aware that she had this on her mind. She merely expressed her random thoughts, and this was what came out.

That the patient was alluding to the therapist in speaking of the clergyman is, of course, an inference, but one supported by experience. It would also seem that she not only considered the possibility that the therapist might be like the clergyman, but that she proceeded to act as though he were. To be self-sufficient and to maintain a distance, she took over and attempted to be her own therapist.

Why did the patient select this particular image of the therapist? There are, of course, many possibilities. Perhaps the therapist resembled the clergyman in appearance, attitude, behavior, or mannerisms. Or perhaps the patient tended to regard all men with whom she might feel close as being like the clergyman, as persons who would try to use her and who would look down on her. In creating this picture, it is likely that she was responding mainly to her own preconceptions.

In the instance just cited, should the therapist make any comments? By all means! If the patient continues to harbor the notion that she will be used and looked down upon, it will seriously interfere with the development of a good working alliance. The therapist should point out that when she speaks of the clergyman as a person whose own house is not in order, she is expressing her fear that the therapist will be like him.

Another woman had struggled to clarify her preconceptions about the therapist. In this instance, unlike the one just cited in which the connection between her male therapist and another man was inferred, the patient made the connection herself.

> *Ms. J stated that it was difficult for her to speak because the therapist's appearance and manner reminded her of the man to whom she had been engaged, a man who was self-centered and interested in sexual conquests. After recounting experiences to substantiate her claim, she suddenly said, "I just happened to think that I always go to women doctors. There's nothing wrong with me now, but I've been looking for a woman doctor in this city just in case." After a brief silence, she mentioned that it was difficult for her "to get started with a man." It was essential for the man to approach her and take the initiative.*

The patient had begun by commenting on the resemblance of the therapist to one man. Then it occurred to her that she placed all men—even physicians—in the same category, interested in her only for narcissistic and sexual reasons. Still, it was essential that the man approach her and take the initiative. The therapist needed to point out how her reaction to men makes it difficult for her to take the initiative in psychotherapy and be comfortable in working with a male therapist. Not only does calling attention to how past experiences shape present expectations help prevent an impasse, but it also provides a graphic introduction to how psychotherapy works (Hollender 1965).

The Therapist as a Real Person

Thus far the focus has been on the patients' preconceptions in determining their response to the therapist. As mentioned previously, however, it would be a mistake to think of the therapist as the same kind of stimulus as the blank card on the Thematic Apperception Test. Patients may detect marked character traits and react, sometimes intensely, to them. Among these traits may be arrogance and superciliousness, as well as tenderness and compassion. While it would be unreasonable to expect therapists to wear masks and coats of armor, how much or how little of any particular feeling should show is moot. Regardless of how much, however, therapists should be sufficiently aware of their own traits to recognize that the patient's productions are not entirely unprovoked and solely the expression of psychological problems. In responding, the therapist should acknowledge, implicitly or explicitly, the validity of the observations, but on occasion suggest that the reactions evoked may still merit further scrutiny.

Relating to the Patient

Not only do patients respond to the therapist's behavior, but, of course, the therapist also responds to the patient's behavior. For example, a woman who combated her fear of men by being aggressive provoked her therapist, who then took countermeasures. Instead of pointing out how she belittled him, he jabbed back by calling attention to her lack of femininity in attire, mannerisms, and speech. He was vaguely aware of feeling uneasy—the type of signal that should be heeded—but was unable to recognize the source of this feeling until the pattern of attack and counterattack was spelled out for him.

Therapist-Patient Relationship

Like Tower (1956), we simply do not believe that any two persons, regardless of circumstance, can closet themselves in a room, day after day, without something happening to each of them in respect to the other. In every prolonged, close relationship—partnership, friendship, or marriage—inevitably each person's personality impinges on the other, and in everyday life, patients learn from the *behavior* of therapists with whom they meet regularly. Education in psychotherapy is no more limited to verbal interventions than education in college is limited to lectures.

Mores and Values

As Marmor (1962) commented, therapists "whether they like it or not, are inevitably purveyors to their patients of some of the fundamental mores and conventional values of their time and milieu." If impulsive behavior is made the object of scrutiny, the therapist conveys the message that this behavior should change.

And, if the therapist calls attention to the patient's strict, inflexible, and oppressive standard, a similar implicit message is sent. Because patient and therapist share the same mores and values to a large extent, it is usually possible for them to concur on what constitutes a problem. As a consequence psychotherapy can work.

It is noteworthy, too, that therapists select patients for their practice from their own social class. Conversely, patients look for therapists with whom they share similar values. The following statement by Hollingshead and Redlich (1958) bears on this point:

> Modern psychotherapy is most likely to succeed when communication is relatively easy between the therapist and patient. Optimal conditions prevail when the therapist and the patient belong to the same social class. All too often, psychotherapy runs into difficulties when the therapist and patient belong to different classes. In these instances, the values of the therapist are too divergent from those of the patient, and communication becomes difficult between them.

Sharing the same mores and values makes it possible for patient and therapist to agree readily on what constitutes problems and how they might be approached, but sharing the same mores and values may also increase the likelihood that ethnic scotoma will constrict the area open to scrutiny and change. Addressing this subject, Shapiro and Pinsker (1973) stated,

> When patient and therapist share the same values and background, the erroneous beliefs or prejudices that they share may be ego syntonic to both and therefore not accessible to analytic scrutiny. The patient who seeks a therapist who "understands" his background is often looking for one who will agree that certain events or attitudes need not be explored or explained, but who will accept them as understandable, i.e., inevitable, consequences of the environment. . . . The therapist who shares his patient's origins may accept without question that which should be analyzed.

The Therapist as a Person

The impact of the therapist as a person certainly is not limited to verbal interventions; it is created in considerable measure by the particular kind of life experience provided and by the values for which he or she stands, or at least seems to stand. Provided by the therapist, too, are understanding, attention, friendliness, warmth, tolerance (in some matters), and helpfulness.

Relatively little has been written concerning the effect of the therapist's personality on the patient, and yet there are reasons, in addition to those cited above, which suggest that personality is of considerable significance. Professionals selecting a therapist to treat a relative or friend, after first excluding those they regard as technically incompetent, are likely to make their choice on the basis of personality factors. In other words, they select the therapist who will offer the type of human relationship they believe the prospective patient seeks and/or needs.

Middle-aged or elderly therapists are able, without upsetting the patient, to make statements that would be upsetting if they came from a younger person. Experience as well as age may account for the difference. For example, older therapists likely can be more casual and matter of fact in discussing sexual topics and under less pressure to be all-knowing in discussing other topics. They can therefore speak more easily and comfortably, with the tone of their voice reflecting a quiet confidence. As a result, like kindly fathers or mothers, they can make statements that might be jarring or threatening if spoken by a younger therapist. On the other hand, a young therapist's energy and enthusiasm may be regarded as just the qualities needed by an older or jaded patient.

The Therapist's Gender

Whether a therapist is a man or a woman may be given undue weight by both patients and those professionals who refer them for therapy. For private patients there is not likely to be a problem; for clinic patients assigned a therapist, there may be a problem. As a general rule, if a prospective patient expresses a strong preference, it should be granted. At the outset of treatment, there are so many possible anxiety-producing circumstances that it is generally wise to do anything that will reduce the distress. Moreover, it is true that some patients initially can establish a better rapport with either a man or a woman. This initial advantage, however, is often offset by the disadvantage of not having the more direct opportunity of working through the difficulty of relating to the person of the nonpreferred gender. For example, a man who has intense anxiety concerning his feelings of competition with other men might prefer a woman therapist, but the result may be that it takes longer for his conflict to become manifest in the transference relationship. For some patients it is productive, after much ground has been covered, to switch from a therapist of one sex to a therapist of the other sex.

The Therapist's Gratification

To round out the picture that has been drawn, it should be added that not only does the therapist influence the patient, but the patient also influences the therapist. In discussing this subject, Tower (1956) stated, "Perhaps the development of a major change in the one, which is, after all, the purpose of the therapy would be impossible without at least some minor change in the other." In other words, the therapist learns something about himself or herself and is influenced by the relationship to the patient, at least to a minor degree.

Therapists should recognize that they derive substantial satisfactions from their work with patients. As Szasz commented, "The medical profession (in common with other authority groups) has a long tradition of denying its own satisfactions and emphasizing its altruistic motives" (Szasz 1956). This attitude, if it makes the patient feel obligated, places a burden on him or her.

Szasz added,

> [W]e have ample reason to believe that an acknowledgment of the analyst's psychological satisfactions in his work—in a fashion which is more explicit and candid than what appears to be the general custom at present—would be desirable for the optimally unhindered psychological development of the analysand. . . . We must remember that in the absence of such a candid appraisal of the analytic situation, there is no safeguard against the hazard of the patient reexperiencing in his relationship with the analyst a human interaction significantly similar to that between a child and a masochistic, "self-sacrificing" parent. (Szasz 1956)

The Nontransference Relationship

In discussing this topic, Greenson and Wexler (1969) stated, "All transference contains some germ of 'reality' and all 'real' relationships have some transference elements." A case was cited in which the patient, in analysis with Greenson, stated, "You always talk a bit too much. You tend to exaggerate. It would be much easier for me to get mad at you. . . . It's terribly hard to say what I mean because I know it will hurt your feelings." Greenson acknowledged that the patient had correctly perceived some traits of his and he added, "It was indeed somewhat painful for me to have them pointed out." He conjectured,

> If the analyst had ignored his [the patient's] remarks, and treated them merely as free associations, or as clinical data to be analyzed, it might have confirmed the patient's feeling that the analyst was too upset to deal with the remarks quite humanly and forthrightly, thereby damaging the working alliance.

Greenson and Wexler (1969) concluded,

> Acknowledging and dealing with nontransference elements need not preclude or obscure the clarification and interpretation of transference. On the contrary, it is our belief that only the development of a viable, "real," nontransference relationship, no matter how limited in scope it may be, is essential to effect the resolution of the transference.

The nontransference relationship may also operate strictly at an unconscious level. For example, a female patient may respond to the feeling that her male therapist finds her attractive without consciously registering the fact. If she struggles with low self-esteem, this response may exert a positive influence. It would be a mistake to assume that nontransference relationships of this kind are uncommon in psychotherapy or that they are only of limited importance. The human responses on the part of the therapist are part of the nonverbal interchange in practically every encounter, and they may impede or promote the therapeutic process.

Therapists' belief systems influence how they will relate to their patients. A positive approach, or even enthusiasm, may follow from the assumption that what they are doing is therapeutically meaningful and helpful. What has been said about the physician prescribing himself or herself with his medication also applies to what the therapist provides along with his or her psychotherapy.

Transference

The term *transference* has been used several times above in an effort to define the nontransferential aspects of the therapeutic relationship. Unfortunately, it is a term often used inappropriately. It is important to distinguish the phenomenon of transference from the realistic aspects of interpersonal relationships.

Probably the interpersonal component of psychotherapy, with particular emphasis on transference, is the most important therapeutic agent in insight-oriented psychotherapy.

Freud used his understanding of the phenomenon of transference as a means of relieving the uneasiness engendered in Breuer by the feelings his patient, Anna O, had expressed for him (Hollender 1980). In doing so, he helped Breuer overcome his reluctance to collaborate on a book on hysteria. Following a description of these events, Jones (1953) recounted, "Freud's remark had evidently made a deep impression, since when they were preparing the Studies together, Breuer said apropos of the transference phenomenon, 'I believe that is the most important thing we both have to make known to the world.'" Although this statement was motivated by Breuer's personal feelings, it is nevertheless probably an accurate assessment of the significance of transference for psychotherapy.

Freud (1905a) defined transference as a whole series of psychological experiences which are revived, not as belonging to the past, "but as applying to the person of the physician at the present moment." The following definition has also been suggested: "A patient's transference to the analyst is only that part of the patient's reaction to the analyst which repeats the patient's reactions to a person who has, at some previous time, played an important role in the patient's life" (French 1946).

Transference may be regarded in three ways: 1) as an obstacle to uncovering the unconscious, i.e., a resistance; 2) as a means of uncovering the unconscious; and 3) "as the condition under which it is eminently possible to bring direct influence to bear on the patient" (Waelder 1956).

Transference as a resistance is encountered when the patient instead of remembering the past strives to relive it in a manner more gratifying than it was lived during childhood. He or she makes an effort to evoke particular responses and is reluctant or even unwilling, for a time, to recognize the reaction as transference.

In pointing out the nature of the patient's behavior, analyzing resistances and scrutinizing the influence of the past on feelings in the present, the transference serves as a means of uncovering the unconscious. Often the very heart of the psychotherapeutic endeavor is working with the transference. It is the grounds par excellence for learning to occur with emotional impact. Freud (1940) stated it well when he said that "the patient never forgets again what he has experienced in the form of transference; it has greater force of conviction for him than anything he can acquire in other ways."

Transference reactions are usually reported when they are experienced, whereas most other reactions are reported after a period of time has elapsed. The former is analogous to the marked physiological changes recorded in an experimental situation when the subject is angry at the investigator, whereas the latter is like the relatively small change noted when the subject talks about anger felt sometime in the past. It should be added that the therapist can be most certain of what is happening when it takes place in the transference because the reaction not only occurs in relationship to him or her, but also occurs in his or her full view (Wolstein 1964).

In discussing transference, Holt (1985) stated,

> Thus, if we hypothesize that someone unconsciously hates his father, we cannot be certain that he will have trouble with *all* persons in authority over him or any specific one, or that such trouble will take any particular form, but we can fairly confidently predict that he will behave in one or more ways that make up a describable *class of events* (e.g., "having trouble with authority figures").

It has been maintained that regression (see Chapter 10) is a prerequisite for the development and resolution of the transference neurosis. However, patterns of behavior stemming from the past are always in evidence in the patient's relationship to the therapist and other people. Thus, it is possible to see the old blueprint that shapes the present pattern of behavior without inducing regression. In treatment, the patient learns first about one aspect of the transference and then another.

Transference can serve as the ideal medium for learning, or it can be used for the purpose of exerting influence over patients. Waelder (1956) took the position that the therapist could use the transference to bring direct influence to bear; others contend that the transference should not be used in this manner. Induced regression and positive transference increase the therapist's power over the patient. Both states promote compliance, and in doing so may exert an influence *antithetical* to the goals of education and self-determination. The danger for insight-oriented psychotherapy is that the patient may be prevailed upon to adopt viewpoints that belong to the therapist and that are not really his or her own.

While positive transference has sometimes been left unanalyzed to facilitate the therapeutic process (especially when the goal is to achieve a so-called transference cure), negative transference has almost always been regarded as an obstacle and actively analyzed (see Chapter 12). However, positive transference presents a special danger, the danger that it might be used for Pygmalion-like purposes. To preclude this possibility in insight-oriented psychotherapy, it should be analyzed as energetically as negative transference.

Closely related to the use of the transference to influence the patient is its use to provide direct gratification. The following example illustrates the "good parent" pitfall.

> *A young woman complained that she received little recognition from her parents when she did well in grammar school. The girl next door, in contrast, received much recognition. The therapist remarked that the patient had wanted recognition from him during the previous hour. He added, "I did notice how well you had done." In pointing out the patient's desire for recognition from him, information was provided; in stating that she had done well, he offered direct gratification of the transference wish. Moreover, it was no longer only that the patient felt like a child in relationship to the therapist, but that she was now placed in a child's position in relationship to him.*

It should be borne in mind that the personality of the therapist may influence the nature of the transference to an extent. In this connection Fenichel (1941) stated,

> Different analysts act differently and these differences influence the behavior of patients. Thus, as is well-known, the sex of the analyst plays a role decisive for the character of the transference reactions of many patients. It is remarkable that with other patients the sex of the analyst appears to be quite a matter of indifference.

As it did for Breuer, the transference may assist the therapist in coping with his or her own feelings. If the patient's love and hate are really intended for someone else, they need not be taken personally. By remaining somewhat detached, a comfortable distance is maintained. This position is probably helpful and necessary. There is the danger, however, that the concept of transference will be used like a shield (a defense), and that the therapist, hiding behind it, will fail to see that some thrusts are directed at him or her as a real person and not as a stand-in. For example, if the therapist is high-handed, the patient may respond with anger. This response is provoked in the present and is not based to an appreciable extent on a pattern laid down in the past. If the patient's complaints are never regarded as appropriate for the present circumstance and always ascribed to transference, he or she may feel like a card player in a game with a stacked deck.

There is a wide variety of transference reactions because different people have experienced different relations with others in the past. A patient may see a need to compete with the therapist much as he or she competed with an older sibling in the past, or, there may be a need to idealize the therapist as omnipotent and omniscient, similar to feelings once held in childhood toward parents. Some types of transference may be especially difficult to deal with and/or require specific techniques, for example, a patient with intense sexualized feelings toward the therapist. Such situations are discussed in greater detail in Chapter 14.

Countertransference

Countertransference has been defined in at least three different ways. The term was originally used "to designate the emotional reactions of the analyst to [against] the patient's transference" (Gitelson 1951). Secondly, it has been used "to cover all the feelings which the analyst experiences towards his patient" (Heimann 1950). Thirdly, it has been used for "only those phenomena which are transferences of the analyst to his patient" (Tower 1956). The third definition is the generally accepted meaning of the term today.

In examining countertransference we should ask: Is it always bad—an interference? In this connection, Heimann (1950) stated,

> I have been struck by the widespread belief amongst candidates that the countertransference is nothing but a source of trouble. Many candidates are afraid and feel guilty when they become aware of feelings toward their patients and consequently aim at avoiding any emotional response and at becoming completely unfeeling and "detached."

On the same subject, Tower (1956) stated, "Interactions (or transactions) between the transferences of the patient and the countertransferences of the analyst, going on at unconscious levels, may be—or perhaps always are—of vital significance for the outcome of the treatment." Finally, Reich (1951) maintained,

"Countertransference is a necessary prerequisite of analysis. If it does not exist, the necessary talent and interest is lacking."

> *A young female resident in psychiatry had an elderly depressed woman in treatment. After several sessions the therapist took over and began to give advice and instructions to the patient, who was cognitively intact and competent. The patient responded with increasing anxiety and the feeling that she was being treated as if she was incapable of handling her own affairs.*

In supervision it became apparent that the therapist was reminded unconsciously of her rigid and controlling mother. Her response was that "the best defense is a good offense," and she struck out in a controlling manner. Once aware of what she was doing and the source of her reaction, she was able to alter her approach.

Because countertransferences reflect the role of the therapist's own transferences into the therapeutic situation there is, as for the patient, a wide range of such possibilities. A therapist may respond to a patient as if he or she were a parent, a child, or a sibling, thereby evoking inappropriate interventions. Robertiello and Schoenewolf (1987) have described a wide range of different forms of countertransference reactions and suggested that attention to the concept of countertransference/counterresistance is as important to the therapeutic process as is transference/resistance.

Acknowledgment of Errors

During the course of psychotherapy, a patient may contend that an interpretation is incorrect. If the therapist realizes that an error has been made, the error should be acknowledged. By acknowledgment is meant a brief, direct statement. The inclination, perhaps because of guilt as the consequence of a countertransference reaction, may be to offer an explanation or an apology. Such a response simply burdens the patient with the therapist's problem. Only under special circumstances is an explanation or an apology either appropriate or helpful.

The acknowledgment of a technical error, such as an incorrect interpretation, is a proper and adequate response, but an apology is called for when there has been a lapse in professional behavior, such as forgetting a scheduled appointment, scheduling two patients for the same time, or falling asleep during a session.

The apology should be brief and may be accompanied by an explanation. For example, if the therapist has fallen asleep it may be explained that he or she was awake all night working in the emergency room. The explanation makes the act less personalized and takes the burden of responsibility off the patient.

In writing on this subject, Greenson (1972) stated,

> I believe it is right to apologize to a patient when your behavior has been unnecessarily hurtful. Not to do so is to be disrespectful and impolite. Yet I have heard of psychoanalysts who have fallen asleep during a patient's hour and when awakened by the patient, remained silent or interpreted the event as a result of the patient's wish to put the analyst in a stupor.

Acknowledgment of errors may have a subtle therapeutic effect in that it is a reminder that the therapist is human, not omniscient, and that the ultimate responsibility for the success of therapy rests in considerable measure with the patient.

Summary

As with other interpersonal relationships, each party brings to therapy their experiences from past relationships which both consciously and unconsciously affect the new relationship. Insight-oriented psychotherapy is different from other social relationships, however, in that the therapist is a participant-observer and as such both experiences and interprets the nature of the relationship.

6

Insight-Oriented Psychotherapy: Fundamental Principles and Techniques

The principles and techniques of psychotherapy are designed to ensure that the "insights" developed are derived from the patient's unconscious and not from the therapist's influence over the patient's thinking and behavior. For insight-oriented psychotherapy, the funadamental principle is that the patient maintains responsibility for his or her own life. The therapist, who functions somewhat like a catalyst, helps patients to help themselves and thereby increases their understanding of inner psychic mechanisms. Through such insights autonomous decisions can be made by the patient as to both the need and the direction for change.

Freud recommended that the patient free associate and that the therapist listen with evenly hovering attention and assume a neutral stance. These three objectives sound reasonable and desirable, but when they are scrutinized it quickly becomes apparent that in reality they are as unattainable as a bloodless surgical field.

Neutrality of the Therapist

What is meant by a neutral stance? Surely it is not that therapists should keep their distance and come across as cold, detached, unfeeling, or sphinx-like. Yet, this is how an attempt at neutrality may be perceived. Perhaps what Freud really had in mind in recommending a neutral stance was that therapists should try to avoid being critical, biased, and prejudiced, and above all they should not moralize or inflict their own personal predilections and preferences on their patients. In other words, neutrality is aimed more at describing what therapists should not do than at what they should do.

Marmor (1962) stated,

> One of the most prevalent dogmas in psychoanalysis is the assumption that the psychoanalyst should and can be a neutral figure, a kind of "mirror" who does not interact with the patient but merely reflects the latter's own feelings and thoughts back to him. I would like to offer the suggestion that such neutrality is a fiction; that in the transactional relationship that exists between patient and therapist, the very effort to be impersonal or neutral is an active attitude which must affect the patient either positively or negatively, depending on his needs. In some instances efforts at "neutrality" on the part of the therapist—silence, inactivity, passivity—may be experienced by the patient as reassurance, absence of pressure, and freedom from moral judgment. In other patients, the identical behavior may be experienced as coldness, lack of empathy and even critical rejection.

In describing the qualities of a good therapist, Strupp (1973) stated,

> They [the qualities] are the attributes of a good parent and a decent human being who has a fair degree of understanding of himself and his interpersonal relations so that his own problems do not interfere, who is reasonably warm and empathic, not unduly hostile or destructive, and who has the talent, dedication, and compassion to work cooperatively with others.

He added that the therapist should avoid " 'criticizing,' 'lecturing,' and generally 'getting in the way' " (Strupp 1973).

Free Association

In regard to free association, Freud (1909) stated, "I made him [the patient] pledge himself to submit to the one and only condition of the treatment—namely, to say everything that came into his head, even if it was *unpleasant* to him, or seemed *unimportant* or *irrelevant* or *senseless.*"

Free association was the natural heir to hypnosis and was designed to circumvent or overcome resistance and to uncover repressed memories or unconscious material. Therapists recognized, however, that the instruction to free associate imposed a "rule" that was never fully obeyed. As Spitz (1956) stated, "I am well aware that this is a rule more honored in its breach than in its observance." Moreover, if the rule were fully obeyed, it would lead to an undesirable result because it presupposes relinquishment of self-observation. Further, completely uninhibited free association would prevent a patient from taking the focused approach to specific areas of conflict often necessary for their resolution.

In commenting on this issue, Anna Freud (1936) said,

> Even today many beginners in analysis have an idea that it is essential to succeed in inducing their patients really and invariably to give all their associations without modification or inhibition, i.e., to obey implicitly the fundamental rule of analysis. But even if their ideal were realized, it would not represent an advance, for after all it would simply mean the conjuring-up again of the now obsolete situation of hypnosis, with its one-sided concentration on the part of the physician upon the id. Fortunately for analysis such docility in the patient is in practice impossible.

Thus, although patients are encouraged to speak of whatever comes to mind, they undoubtedly will be selective to an extent and they are likely to exercise their right to be silent. If they do so, the therapist should not step into the breach by suggesting a topic for discussion or making a comment. They may either wait for the patient to begin speaking again or inquire about the patient's thoughts.

Listening and Observing

Freud (1912), in recommending "evenly hovering attention," warned that "as soon as attention is deliberately concentrated in a certain degree, one begins to select from the material." Evenly hovering attention is a type of listening that is relatively nonselective and passive. At times therapists may listen as recommended by Freud but it seems unlikely that they will be able to do so for sustained periods. French (1958) commented that "sooner or later selection cannot be avoided." He added, "If the analyst is trying to anticipate at each point how the patient will react, he will be more alert to recognize the patient's responses when they do occur and then to use them for purposes of demonstration."

As surely as patients will exercise some choice in what they say, therapists will bring a particular point of view and a particular focus to what they hear. To an appreciable degree the therapeutic process will be—and probably should be—selective and active.

As therapists listen, they will be influenced by information gathered previously and especially during the preceding hour. Instead of allowing the material to seep in, an assist may be given to the effort at unconscious processing. This can be done by converting a mass of details into a few main headlines. In other words, a 10- to 15-minute monologue or dialogue can be reduced to a single sentence, summarizing or capturing the essence of it. By doing this with several segments of the hour, the material is converted into workable form. The patient's statements may also be supplemented by other information—for example, a particular interpretation made during the previous hour or the fact, known to the patient, that the therapist will soon leave on vacation.

If at times the therapist's imagination has been permitted to range freely, a hypothesis may be formed that can be subjected to disciplined scrutiny before it is used as the basis for an interpretation. This process is similar to the preliminary stages of a research project: Using imagination, an investigator develops a hypothesis that is then subjected to critical scrutiny to determine if it seems plausible.

To think of the therapist's task as being similar to an intellectual exercise, like adding a column of figures or solving a problem in logic, would be a mistake. It would also be a mistake to think of the manner of listening as a form of reverie. The task, in fact, is more or less a combination of the two, with the weight of each varying from time to time. Although the focus has been on the spoken word as the main currency of psychotherapy, it should be understood that nonverbal communication is also the source of significant information.

The Therapist's Questions

Interpretation (see Chapter 7) may be the hallmark of insight-oriented psychotherapy, but it is by no means the only type of technical intervention. Although asking questions may seem innocuous (and answering questions is commonplace), verbal interchange is highly colored by them. Eissler (1953) stated, "It is doubtful if any person was ever analyzed without being asked questions by the analyst in the course of the psychoanalytic treatment." In all likelihood every analysand is asked many questions.

One of the most common and obvious reasons the therapist asks questions is *to clarify a point.* To minimize ambiguity and to eliminate misapprehensions, there is no substitute for questions.

Another common reason for asking questions is to *elicit additional information* that might be helpful in supporting or excluding a hypothesis being considered as the basis for an interpretation. A third purpose for asking questions is to encourage the patient *to explore a subject* mentioned in passing that might prove to be the source of significant information.

In some circumstances, queries are most effectively made by restating in an interrogative form the last sentence or phrase the patient uttered (Deutsch 1939). This useful technique encourages the patient's train of thought while being minimally disruptive. It is, of course, a form of "positive reinforcement" and, like any other technical intervention, does influence the course of therapy.

Obviously, only questions consistent with the goals of psychotherapy should be raised. Questions that merely satisfy the personal curiosity of the therapist are out of place. The same rule applies to questions that derive from research rather than therapeutic interest.

Besides raising questions anyone would be likely to raise, therapists should feel free to ask questions very few persons would ask. These questions may bring out and dust off cherished but unfounded notions and assumptions. For example, if patients treat their own body with indifference, they might be asked, "Who do you feel your body belongs to—your parents, God, or yourself?" Also, if patients talk of things happening to them, the therapist might ask, "Did they just happen to you or did you do something to make them happen?"

At the same time that questions open some vistas to scrutiny, they close others. Also, to an extent, how questions are worded will build in or block out certain possible answers. Langer (1942) noted, "The 'technique' or treatment, of a problem begins with its first expression as a question. The way a question is asked limits and disposes the ways in which any answer to it—right or wrong—may be given." In asking questions, therapists unavoidably reveal information about their own personal and cultural bias. To expect them to do otherwise would be like expecting a fish to live out of water. Patients will not be unduly influenced, however, if they are free to disagree with the therapist and if their difference of opinion is recognized, accepted, and respected. Most therapists probably do not find it difficult to avoid or circumvent the deep and open pits of personal and cultural bias. For example, if they would inquire why a man was thinking of divorce, they would also inquire why he was thinking of returning to his wife. Questions should, and usually do, examine both sides of an issue. It is the subtle value judgments that are likely to escape notice.

"Why" questions merit special consideration. The therapist may ask why to obtain additional information, but patients may react as though their behavior is being criticized or their motives impugned. Accordingly, they may proceed to attempt to justify their actions. This problem in communication is so common that therapists should constantly be on the alert for it. If signs of it are detected, an immediate effort should be made to abort the misunderstanding by clarifying the matter. On occasion it may be possible and desirable to preclude such a misunderstanding by asking, "Would you talk more about this subject?" instead of asking, "Why?"

As a general rule, why questions should be used sparingly. They often incorrectly imply that patients have, or should have, knowledge of unconscious forces. Thus, they may block a more fruitful and complete investigation of an area. In this regard, "what" or "when" or "how" questions provide for further exploration of the topic at issue, and the "why" emerges as a logical consequence. At times if the therapist does not ask a question, silence seems to signify agreement. For example, if patients speak of themselves in disparaging terms, silence implies that this assessment is shared. Once any question has been asked, silence no longer can be regarded as neutral. Seeming to agree with the patients' self-depreciation engenders an unfriendly or critical atmosphere and results in a poor educational or therapeutic climate.

Therapists should be alert to the possibility of being baited to ask questions. The patient, playing a cat-and-mouse game, may dangle a verbal morsel well chosen to pique curiosity. If therapists respond by raising questions, they will fall into the trap of playing the cat-and-mouse game instead of helping the patient learn why this particular game is played. An interpretation, and not a question, is in order. The following rule of thumb should be kept in mind: *It is more pertinent to find out why the patient behaves coyly or experiences difficulty in continuing to speak than to extract or discern what is being suppressed.*

The Patient's Questions

Questions the therapist asks are on one side of the ledger; on the other side are the questions the patient asks. The response to the patient's questions may be 1) silence, 2) a direct answer, 3) a question such as "Why do you ask?" or "What do you think?" 4) a direct answer followed by the query "Why do you ask?" or 5) an interpretation. To a considerable extent, the response depends on what is understood as the reason for the question.

Obviously, some questions should be taken at face value. Examples are an inquiry to determine if an appointment time can be changed because of an unavoidable scheduling problem and a request for information about the date that the therapist will leave on vacation. Questions like these come up infrequently, and even then the possibility of a hidden meaning should not be overlooked.

In some instances, a direct answer is most appropriate.

A young man asked his therapist how she could say that the picture he presented of his wife was out of balance. She responded, "You pick out something to complain about in everything she does, even in the instances which you preface with the words 'I must admit.' Then, after grudgingly admitting that she occasionally does something to please you, you even cancel that out."

With questions other than those asked for obvious reasons, the therapist's principal concern should be "Why is the question asked?" If the therapist believes that he or she knows, optimally the response should be in the form of an interpretation.

The following account of an hour illustrates how a patient's questions may be handled.

A young man who had been in treatment for several months opened an hour by commenting on his first significant sexual experience. The experience had occurred recently and had been only partially successful from his standpoint. He then mentioned that he was thinking of two questions he wished to ask but was reluctant to do so because he was sure the therapist would inquire why he asked. The first question was "Had you [the therapist] gone to medical school with the intention of becoming a psychiatrist?" The second questions was "Were you originally from the city in which you received your training?" The patient added that he would find it difficult to understand why anyone would move from a large city to a smaller one. Both questions were answered in a few words.

The patient next acknowledged another bit of curiosity about the therapist by stating that he thought of hiding near the front entrance of the office building to see what kind of car the therapist drove. He pictured the therapist in a Cadillac. At this point it was suggested that the patient's curiosity ran deeper than his questions might at first indicate. He smiled and said, "It's probably something sexual." When asked what he thought the car referred to, he replied, "Something phallic." He laughed uncomfortably and then stated that in the shower room lately he found himself constantly comparing the size of his penis with those of other men. He explained that his genital development had been somewhat delayed and that at high school he had been embarrassed when he undressed in the locker room because his classmates poked fun at him. He added that he was proud of the size of his penis now. It was pointed out that his curiosity stemmed from his interest in comparing the size of his penis with that of his therapist. Although his penis was large now, in his mental picture it was still small. This was similar to the general picture he had of himself. Although he was now tall, he still tended to think of himself as short whenever he entered a new situation. (He had mentioned this reaction approximately 25 hours earlier in speaking of his late growth spurt.)

The patient's questions and his fantasy (of hiding to see the therapist's car) pointed to a specific, but unconscious, type of curiosity. His wish to compare his manliness with his therapist's manliness was a reaction to being only partially successful in his recent sexual experience and the reactivation of the picture of himself as an underdeveloped little boy who felt inadequate in comparison to his peers and father.

A special question is "What do you think of me?" This question is special because it goes to the heart of self-esteem. Although usually raised indirectly, occasionally it is asked in so many words. The following instance is one in which the patient gradually zeros in on the target.

A patient opened the hour by commenting on how well she had parked her car. She then asked the therapist what he thought about her progress in treatment. Also, she wanted to know what diagnosis he had written on her clinic chart. She explained that when her otolaryngologist examined her sinuses, he let her know if they looked good or bad. She added, "I hope you don't see what he saw. The last time he looked, he said, 'Ugh.'" Like a camera moving in for a closeup, she proceeded on and asked, "What do you think of me?" It might be pointed out that she had called attention to

> *how well she had done and then quite naturally wished to be commended. At the same time she seemed concerned that something might be found beneath the surface (or inside) that would evoke a critical "Ugh."*

Although the focus is on understanding a question as part of a message, requests for information should not regularly be met with stony silence. At times the patient should be reminded of the therapist's interest in why a question is posed. It is sometimes appropriate, too, for the therapist to state that he or she does not know the answer to a particular question but will try to help find it.

Summary

Several fundamental principles and techniques of insight-oriented psychotherapy that appear to be remarkably simple have been presented. On closer scrutiny these ground rules are fundamental and facilitate the unfolding of unconscious mental processes. They also presuppose values that emphasize respect for individual differences and self-determination.

7

Insight-Oriented Psychotherapy: Technical Interventions

Of the various technical operations in insight-oriented psychotherapy, the most distinctive is the interpretation. Through it the therapist's understanding of the patient's unconscious mental processes are conveyed to patients. In addition to interpretations, other technical interventions available to therapists include comments, summaries, recapitulations, confrontations, and acknowledgments.

Interpretations

An interpretation is an informative statement based on decoding the patient's communication. It serves to bring unconscious content into consciousness. As such it adds to the patient's self-knowledge. In this respect it contrasts with the informative comments (to be discussed later) from which information may be gained but not of the unconscious dimension.

The interpretation most clearly differentiates psychotherapy from everyday conversation. In social situations one person does not ordinarily decode the hidden meaning of a message for the other person. In psychotherapy, however, doing so is an essential part of the therapeutic process. As French (1958) emphasized, two steps are usually involved in preparation for an interpretation. The first step is reaching a hypothesis about the patient's unconscious communication, and the second is deciding if the information should be imparted to the patient and, if so, in what form.

The process of listening and hypothesis-formation can be likened to an internist taking a patient's history for the purpose of making a diagnosis. In the medical situation the patient's first complaint may be as general as "I hurt; I'm in pain." At this point there are innumerable possible diagnoses. If the next bit of information is that the pain is in the chest, the number of possible diagnoses is greatly reduced. And when it is learned that other symptoms include cough with a rusty sputum and chills and fever, the working diagnosis is narrowed down to one.

Much as the acumen of the internist is taxed by vague or poorly defined symptoms, the acumen of the therapist will be challenged by veiled communications. And just as the correct diagnosis will be made only if the internist considers a particular disease as a possibility, so an interpretation that fits will be found only if the therapist considers a particular hypothesis.

The therapist, in going through a process similar to the one described for the internist, may reach a single hypothesis that can serve as the basis for an interpretation. This process is illustrated by the following clinical note of a treatment hour.

> *A young man, Mr. E, opened an hour with the statement that his feelings toward work and his general outlook on life varied from day to day. The variability he ascribed to something physical, perhaps metabolic. This opening statement, like the complaint of pain, allows for innumerable possibilities.*
>
> *Mr. E then mentioned that he had encountered several business problems on a particular day. After enumerating them, he described each one in detail. To this exposition, two facts were added. The first was that the "particular day" to which he referred was Tuesday, and the second was that he wondered if his therapist would be more concerned about him if he caused as much trouble as some of his customers caused him. The therapist had canceled Mr. E's Tuesday appointment. The following hypothesis was now tenable: Mr. E struggled to maintain the idea that his feelings and outlook were the product of physical, and hence impersonal, factors. By doing so he denied the likelihood that he felt bad because the therapist had been away and he missed him.*
>
> *Based on this hypothesis, the therapist suggested that it was not Mr. E's metabolism but the canceled appointment that was responsible for the way he felt. Mr. E responded, "I wondered why you took the day off." He quickly added that he did not mean to express himself the way it sounded; he assumed the therapist had important business that probably took him out of town. Moreover, he had been away himself on business from time to time. It was pointed out that although he tried to be logical and unemotional in viewing the situation, perhaps the way he really felt was expressed in the comment that the therapist had taken the day off.*

Mr. E then suggested that the therapist must have to work harder with disturbed patients. In response the therapist stated that Mr. E felt he was taken for granted because he was so conforming and well-behaved; that people who were less conforming and less well-behaved received more attention. This interpretation led to the recollection of how he envied a childhood friend who always stirred up trouble. The patient could not afford to be like his friend, so he believed, because he had less ability and talent. Moreover, at home not only was he expected to be conforming, but compliance was well rewarded (Hollender 1965).

Decoding Unconscious Communications

As the patient speaks, the therapist listens and simultaneously scans the content and the nonverbal messages against the backdrop of the patient's past history, defensive structure, and relationship with the therapist. Information that does not appear relevant may suddenly become meaningful if the form in which it is presented can be decoded.

Simple code forms. Relatively simple or transparent messages consist of a single statement or brief story and often are readily decoded. One patient spoke of how critical his wife was of the therapist. He mentioned this at a time when it could be inferred he himself was also critical of the therapist. Moreover, his pattern was to impute feelings to others when he found it difficult to express them himself. A rhetorical question such as "Who feels so critical?" could serve as a "clarification interpretation" (Colby 1951).

Complex code forms. Complex messages may be composed of parts that seem unrelated. With these longer narratives (as in the case of Mr. E previously cited), special attention should be paid to the juxtaposition of ideas. By doing so it may be possible to identify an internally consistent thesis to account for what seem on the surface to be *non sequiturs.* In other words, in these instances, the connections may be found in the unconscious.

To offer a comprehensive or more or less complete interpretation, it is necessary to identify the precipitant, the reaction it evokes, the reason it causes a conflict, and the manner in which the conflict is addressed. This approach is illustrated by the following excerpts from two consecutive hours.

> *During the first hour, Mrs. F spoke of feelings of hostility that seemed especially intense. The next hour she stated that she had exerted much control over her behavior, and she referred to the hostility mentioned during the previous hour. She was also aware of eating more and of putting on weight. She next made some comments about a physician who reduced a woman's number of monthly visits because she could not afford his regular fee. The woman did not feel free to complain or express anger because she felt so indebted to the physician for help he had given her in the past. At this point the therapist reminded the patient that her visits had recently been reduced in number. She objected to the implication that this had anything to do with her reaction of intense hostility, pointing out that she had requested the reduction in hours. However, when it was suggested that perhaps she felt that the therapist should not have acceded to her request, she agreed that the change might have been the precipitant of her reaction.*
>
> *The pattern now seemed clear. The reduction in hours had mobilized hostility that the patient was afraid would jeopardize her relationship with the therapist. Moreover, she felt too indebted to him for help he had given her to complain or express anger. She therefore held back her feelings and in particular attempted to control her hostility. As a result she cut herself off from gratification she might have derived in interpersonal relationships. She then turned to food as a substitute. Finally, she recognized that her current reactions recapitulated an old pattern with her mother.*

Aids to decoding. Three aids will be discussed, the first of which can be regarded as *alerters* and consists of qualifying remarks such as "It probably doesn't mean anything but I'll tell you about it anyway . . . " and "It's not important but. . . . " Such disclaimers often precede statements that are emotionally charged and quite revealing. Thus, these remarks and others like them telegraph the message "Listen attentively." They must alert even the therapist attempting to maintain evenly hovering attention.

"Doorknob remarks" are statements a patient makes on the way out of the office. Although these statements are voiced casually, they may be especially revealing because they are emitted at an off-guard moment. Not all doorknob remarks, however, are expressions of a relaxation of censorship; some merely are a last-minute attempt to divulge something previously withheld or to clarify an issue.

A second aid to decoding might be labeled the *organizing piece.* It refers to an event in the patient's life or in therapy that should be known by the person who works to unravel the meaning of a message. The event might not be momentous by ordinary standards, but it takes on special significance because it plays into old feelings. The current circumstance that mobilizes old feelings of rejection or loss may be a canceled appointment, an approaching vacation, or a reduction in the number of hours of therapy. With the organizing piece in mind, it may be easy to decode a message; without it, the message may seem to consist of several unrelated parts.

A third aid might be labeled *continuity and context.* Because there is *continuity* from one hour to the next, unless an outside intercurrent event of considerable magnitude is interposed, it is important for therapists to refresh their memory about the major theme of the previous hour before beginning the next session.

Not only is there likely to be continuity from hour to hour, with the opening statement of one hour following the closing statement of the previous hour as though no time elapsed in between, but also during a cluster of hours psychodynamic themes can be expected to emerge. These themes often follow familiar patterns. For instance, a young woman may be coy and seductive to elicit attention and interest from men (and this may include the therapist) to help combat a poor self-image. Her objective is not to have a sexual relationship. Only later will her sexuality come into focus. (There is the danger, in therapy and elsewhere, that her coy and seductive behavior will be misread as a primary interest in sex.)

The following is another example: When assertiveness and aggressiveness, so often associated with masculinity in our culture, are inhibited, the result is a feminine self-concept. Because of shame, this self-concept is hidden behind a pseudo-masculine facade. In therapy, the theme evolves in the following sequence: 1) pseudo-masculine facade (machismo), 2) feminine self-concept, and 3) fear of expressing "masculine" assertiveness and aggressiveness (Alexander 1933).

The two themes presented as examples, and others like them, provide a *context* within which each hour fits. This overview makes it possible to see where the various parts belong in the larger story. A word of caution, however, is necessary. There is the danger that the guidelines suggested, if followed too rigidly, will be responsible for forcing patients into preformed molds.

In addition to aids to decoding, there are *special signals,* signals to make the therapist aware that something is amiss. For example, a patient may hint that the therapist is not grasping the meaning of a message by talking about people who miss the point of a story. Similar allusions may appear in dreams.

Types of Interpretations

Interpretations are of two basic types: 1) *content* and 2) *meta. Content* interpretation refers to a statement based on the substance of the message. *Meta* interpretation refers to the form in which a message is presented. Content is concerned with *what* is said; meta is concerned with *how* it is said. For example, if patients speak of highly moving events as though they were commenting on the weather, the emotional detachment and the reason for it—probably the need to fend off feelings—should be pointed out before or instead of interpreting the content of the message.

A meta interpretation may include more than a statement about the tone of voice or the nature of mannerisms. For example, a patient who wishes to become self-determining may still be so intent on pleasing the therapist that he or she works more diligently at it than at acquiring self-knowledge. The patient is like the student who relinquishes his or her personal strivings to please the teacher. This maneuver, not the content, needs to be interpreted.

Presentation of Interpretations

The manner of presentation and the wording of interpretations must suit the therapist. Consequently, much variation is to be expected. No matter what the therapist's style, however, it should be tailored to meet the needs of the particular patient. Just as therapists speak differently to each of their friends, they should speak somewhat differently to each patient, and depending on circumstances they may be wordy or curt, gentle or sharp.

Because the therapist's manner of speaking may convey empathy, interest, and warmth, there is the danger that patients may react more to the feelings than to the content of the messages. Probably there is no way to avoid this, nor need there be. The alternative might be for the therapist to function like a machine ejecting words. In contrast to the warm and friendly approach, this approach would likely be experienced as cold and unfriendly.

The keynote of the therapist's affective response should be *naturalness.* By naturalness is meant responding in a manner consistent with one's own personality. Of course, the response should also be in keeping with the requirements of the therapeutic situation and the patient's particular circumstance. The prevailing interpersonal atmosphere for optimal learning should be that of friendliness, but friendliness should not be construed to mean a friendship.

The language in which an interpretation is presented should be vivid; the words chosen ideally should create a picture and touch the emotions. Pointing out a "sour grapes" attitude or a "Cinderella" fantasy conveys a vivid message. Select words that are precise. For example, to say that a patient is angry may be correct but not precise. It might be more on target to describe the feeling as "spiteful," "petulant," or "vindictive" or to say the patient is having a "temper tantrum." To be petulant or to have a temper tantrum is to be angry in a childish way and therefore might evoke a feeling of shame in an adult. To be merely angry, however, might be passed off without a ripple of discomfort.

Often other important distinctions are not taken seriously enough. It is one thing to want to be a bride, another to be a wife, and one thing to want to bear children, another to be a mother. There is a crucial difference, too, between assertiveness, which means standing one's ground, and aggressiveness, which involves striking out at someone.

As with every generalization, there are exceptions to the rejoinder that words ideally should create a picture and touch the emotions. An exception is the interpretation presented to a sensitive patient who is highly volatile and bounces from one emotional peak to the next. Cold or intellectual language may help such a patient achieve sufficient detachment to deal with the interpretation.

Ideally, an interpretation should contain a single thought. Many rich ideas, like the best answers on an examination, can be stated in a few words or in a sentence or two. Complicated statements may be unclear, as in the following example: "It is also possible that you might not have been trying to get even with your father, but rather you were attempting to become closer to him in a way which was available to you at this time even though it meant punishing yourself." Stated more simply: "Perhaps you hurt yourself to get your father's attention."

The presentation of interpretations may be couched in tentative or positive terms. Tentative ones are introduced by expressions such as "Let me suggest . . . ," "It would seem . . . ," or simply "Possibly . . . " or "Perhaps. . . . " They may even be worded as questions, beginning with "Do you think . . . ?" (When positive interpretations are expressed as questions, the questions are usually rhetorical.) In discussing this subject, Colby (1951) stated,

> Of course, besides the verbal form, the therapist's accompanying tone of voice, gestures and facial expression . . . carry an impact. This is an area uncharted by rules. One principle of help to the beginner is that he should interpret by and large in the form of questions or suggestions, avoiding brandishing his ideas with an air of finality.

With patients who are ready to accept as factual whatever their therapist says, it is especially important to present interpretations in tentative form. On the other hand, with patients who accept nothing unless it makes good sense to them, it is not necessary to be as tentative or cautious.

Because nonverbal responses are part of the message to be decoded, they should be mentioned in connection with an interpretation. For example, a young woman showed intense feelings when she spoke of the "horrible way" an uncle treated his daughter. An interpretation was preceded by a comment about the intense feelings she showed. It was then pointed out that she identified with her cousin and that her uncle's behavior reminded her of how her father treated her when she was a little girl.

The following clinical note illustrates an interpretation made largely in response to a nonverbal communication.

> *A young woman who had come to her first nine appointments wearing a beret that only partly covered a mop of messy hair, came to her tenth appointment with her hair cut and combed. An interpretation (suggested also by what she said) was made that the change in her appearance reflected a change in her feelings about herself.*

The presentation of an interpretation may also be preceded by calling attention to the selection of some words and the avoidance of others. For example, a patient may state repeatedly "One thinks . . . " or "One does . . . " instead of "I think . . . " or "I do. . . . " A patient may refer to a spouse as "my husband (or wife)" instead of using the spouse's first name (or nickname). The interpretation, based on these usages, might be that particular words are chosen in an effort to keep certain feelings muted.

An interpretation may also encompass contradictory statements or mixed messages. One message may be verbal and the other nonverbal, one conscious and the other unconscious. For example, an ace relief pitcher wears number 13 on his jersey, showing that he is not superstitious, but he crosses himself before beginning his warm-up throws. And there is the woman with a plunging neckline who wears a cross in the center of her cleavage.

Timing of Interpretations

Every raconteur knows the importance of timing, and every therapist should also. Well-timed interpretations, like well-timed punch lines, are likely to evoke the desired response. If the therapist always waits for the patient to "run down" or become silent before making an interpretation, the propitious moment may slip away. Occasionally, it is technically—even if not socially—proper for the therapist to interrupt the patient in the interest of optimal effectiveness.

There are ideal times in the course of therapy to make interpretations. A premature interpretation at best is ignored and may be made again at a more appropriate time; at the worst it increases resistance. At the other extreme, an interpretation that has been delayed so long that the message is already known by the patient has failed to advance therapy as rapidly as might be desirable.

Under some circumstances, the timing of an interpretation alters the message. For instance, when a patient is told that he is attracted to a young woman because she resembles his mother, the implication is that he should inhibit sexual impulses toward her as he would toward his mother. On the other hand, if the therapist waits until the patient begins to react with guilt to his sexual impulses and then points out that he does so because he identifies the woman with his mother, the reminder that she is not his mother should reduce his feeling of guilt (Alexander and French 1946).

Responses to Interpretations

It has been said that an interpretation opens a chapter but never closes one. This being the case, it is especially important to know the nature of the effect that has been achieved. How was the interpretation understood? Was it emotionally meaningful? These two questions should be answered, preferably by the patient. Patients who have characteristic patterns of response may be easy to read. When an interpretation clicks, an involuntary smile or a comment like "I see" or "I never thought of it that way" is typical. Some patients look as though they have had a revelation or an uncanny experience. Others react as though they have been caught off guard or found out. There are many patterns;, but each patient is likely to respond in keeping with his or her own personal style.

In the following clinical excerpt, the first interpretation missed the target but the second one hit it.

> *A young man recounted a fantasy of overhearing his therapist comment on his many talents to his employer. The therapist suggested that the patient wanted recognition from both his employer and his therapist. A period of silence was followed by a not very convincing, "I guess so." A subsequent interpretation to the effect that the patient wished that the therapist would intercede for him with his employer, like his father had interceded with his teachers, brought forth a characteristic response.*

In the following instance, the confirmation of the correctness of an interpretation was contained within an immediate, spontaneous retort.

> *A young woman opened an hour by stating that she felt smug and virtuous because she had not acted impulsively the night before. Later she appeared to be upset and said she was almost too embarrassed to continue to speak. She explained that it was because of something sexual. She added, "I was thinking of you stroking my hair—nothing more than that. I'm making our relationship sexual." To this the therapist responded, "You want me to pat you on the head." She laughed and acknowledged, "I want you to be pleased with how well I behaved last night."*

In this instance, the therapist was aware of the patient's predilection to conceal her childish longings behind "adult" sexual behavior. Consequently, like a decoder familiar with a particular code, he quickly and almost automatically read the message. The patient, in turn, had become sufficiently aware of her own pattern of behavior that she immediately confirmed the correctness of the interpretation. The interpretation and the acknowledgment had a ping-pong quality. This type of exchange might be expected when two persons have worked together long enough to become familiar with each other's style (Hollender 1965).

A frequent response to an interpretation is a period of silence. Silence in itself neither confirms nor denies the correctness of an interpretation. However, it probably is a more common response to an incorrect interpretation. Greenson (1961) suggested that silence usually indicates the disappointment in not being understood." When silence follows an "Aha!" reaction that comes with a new insight, it is usually used to mull over the experience.

Thus far, the focus has been on the immediate response to an interpretation. Subsequent responses may be equally significant as is demonstrated by the following example.

> *A woman reacted with intense anger when her husband attended a Christmas party at his office. Because they were Orthodox Jews, she regarded his behavior as unacceptable. She recognized that her stand was strong and perhaps rigid. When it was suggested that her intense reaction stemmed in part from her envy of Christians and their holiday, she first protested saying that she liked her own holidays. After expostulating for at least 10 minutes, she suddenly became silent and then stated that she recalled a childhood experience which suggested to her that the therapist's interpretation might be correct. Her memory was of being invited to share in some festivities of the season with a Christian neighbor. She recalled her attraction to the Christmas tree and the gaiety and warmth pervading the home. For some reason, she continued, she had not thought of this occasion for many years. Evidently her husband, in attending a Christmas party, revived this memory and the envy associated with it that she had kept repressed (Hollender 1965).*

In this instance, both the protest and the memory were responses to the interpretation. Such responses may be followed by other developments, along similar lines, during subsequent hours. An interpretation that fits is like a key that unlocks a storage chest, providing access to what is inside—first the objects on top and then those that are underneath.

During an hour, the therapist sizes up the situation as quickly as possible and makes the interpretation that seems most timely and appropriate. Following the hour, the therapist may mull over what transpired much as one might look at the rerun of a videotape. Learning is fostered in this manner, whether the reviewing is done on one's own or with a supervisor.

Hours Without Interpretations

Clinical experience indicates it is not likely that interpretations will be made in every hour. In hours without interpretations, interchanges may occur in the form of questions and answers and as comments. There are times, however, when the therapist has said little or nothing. In such instances, it is in order to take the advice offered by Greenson and Wexler (1969): "We have found it useful before the end of an hour to tell a patient when we were unclear about what has been going on in the hour. We do not dismiss a patient in silence or reach wildly for some remote interpretation to demonstrate a comprehension we do not have." A statement to the patient like the following might be appropriate: "Perhaps we will soon gain a better understanding of what you are struggling with. Your thoughts about it should prove helpful." The last half of the statement is designed, of course, to encourage the patient's active participation.

Comments

If *interpretations* are the thoroughbreds of psychotherapy, *informative comments* are the workhorses (Hollender 1965). Comments may be of several types, with the major positive ones being described as informative. In addition to informative comments, which have a direct effect on the psychotherapeutic process, other types of comments exert an indirect effect by helping to maintain a favorable climate. Finally, some comments exert an adverse effect by interfering with the work at hand.

Types of Comments

Informative comments. These comments delineate or describe patterns of behavior or aspects of them. Examples are the patients' inability to be assertive or the expectation that they will perform perfectly or their need to please others even if it entails depriving themselves. The list of possibilities is long.

Informative comments also serve to point out the similarities in disparate ideas, events, or circumstances. For example, a patient's attention could be called to the fact that he or she has the same problem in reconciling love and sex as in reconciling religion and evolution. Informative comments may call attention to the nature of reactions or underscore reactions that the patients themselves have detected. The therapist might point out that a patient becomes dizzy in situations in which he or she might have become angry but does not. Or the therapist may point out that the patient's feeling of fatigue is actually an expression of boredom and that a particular feeling labeled depression is actually an expression of unhappiness. If the comment seems plausible to the patient, the subject can be discussed further.

Informative comments may suggest that patients take a new look at themselves or at particular events. They are encouraged to reexamine their attitude and to develop a different perspective. For example, the therapist, after listening to the dramatic recital of several unhappy but seemingly trivial events, may merely say, "So?" This terse expression, implying that too much is made of too little, may be more effective than a lengthy paragraph. The emphasis is on the description of how the patient reacts. Obviously this one-word rejoinder may drive home the point for one patient, but shatter another. As with interpretations, tact and timing are critical.

Informative comments do not go beyond the clinical data and are essentially phenomenological-descriptive in nature. Unlike interpretations, they are not concerned with the unconscious dimension. They often precede interpretations, and in so doing they prepare the way for the more definitive type of intervention. However, to regard them only as stage-setters would be to overlook the intrinsic values they possess and the important role they play.

In addition to serving as a descriptive statement, an informative comment also conveys an implicit message that a particular reaction or pattern may be the cause of some difficulty and therefore should be scrutinized, understood, and changed. An example is the patient who tends to see everything in terms of black or white. In pointing out this pattern, the implicit message is "Why is there no gray?" or even "You should try to find some gray."

Informative comments, like some questions, may be heard as criticism. The following is an example: To the therapist's comment "You keep things very general," the patient responded that she probably did so because she was unable to think clearly. She thought she was being criticized—told she was inadequate or even stupid. Of course, she may have preferred to think she was functioning poorly rather than struggle to cope with troublesome feelings. From a technical standpoint, the first step is to acquaint the patient with her reaction to the comment. This is accomplished by pointing out that she took it as criticism. The therapist's statement invites her to consider why she reacted as she did. Implicit is the message "You misconstrued the meaning of what I said." The second step is to suggest that the reason the patient tends to speak in generalities instead of specifics is to maintain her distance from certain feelings. This adds "why" to "how"—an interpretation to a comment.

Another example is that of a young woman who was extremely self-deprecating and self-critical. When these qualities were pointed out, her immediate response was that these were obviously more of her faults that needed attention. The therapist's next comment was to note that her response was self-deprecating and self-critical. She was embarrassed but acknowledged that this was true. After several sessions she was able to stop herself when she made a self-derogatory statement, acknowledge what she was doing, and then proceed in a less critical manner.

After making an informative comment, it is essential to clarify the nature of the problem to be explored. A person who has been apprehended attempting to swindle a customer may not wish to work on overcoming this antisocial behavior. He merely may want to learn how to operate so that he will not be apprehended again (Horney 1950). In this instance the patient and therapist did not subscribe to the same value system and hence did not agree on the objective of treatment.

Comments as human responses. These comments include the expression of condolence at the death of a family member, good wishes on the birth of a child, or congratulations on graduation from school. Human responses are essential for maintaining a comfortable therapeutic climate. Without such responses the therapist is perceived as cold, unfeeling, and even unreal. Under these circumstances the patient is likely to feel disillusioned or disappointed and angry.

Addressing this issue, Greenson (1972) stated, "I do not greet a patient after a six-week vacation as though I had seen him yesterday. Nor would I end the last hour before a lengthy vacation as though I would see the patient tomorrow." The generalization can be made that if therapists err in one direction, it should be toward being too human.

Extremely anxious patients find prolonged periods of silence difficult to endure, especially during the early phase of treatment. To relieve tension the therapist may interject some comments, however brief and bland. As soon as possible, however, the reaction to silence should be handled in a more definitive manner.

Nonverbal comments. Comments of this kind include facial expressions, body movements, and emitted sounds. Facial expressions may range from a quizzical look to grimacing. Bodily movements may consist of a shrug of the shoulders, making a fist, or cupping an ear. Sounds indicating either understanding or puzzlement are often heard. Nonverbal comments may communicate that the therapist is listening and follows what is being said, believes that a subject should be developed more fully, or does not understand a message. Mandler and Kaplan (1956) and Krasner (1958) have shown that the therapist's "mm-hmms" can be used to manipulate the content of the patient's spontaneous communications. For example, if the therapist says "mm-hmm" every time the past is mentioned and is silent when statements are made about the present, in a short while the patient will begin to talk considerably more about the past than the present. If now the "mm-hmms" are shifted to the present, the content of the communications will be reversed. Thus, the cues act like a reward-punishment operant conditioning system. The communication and behavior of which the therapist approves is reinforced and that of which the therapist disapproves is discouraged. These findings are also relevant to note-taking and other types of behavior that will be discussed later.

Intrusive comments. Comments made without a specific purpose in mind tend to convert an educational and therapeutic endeavor into everyday conversation. The greatest danger is that a chatty comment leading nowhere will be made when an interpretation might have had a more telling effect.

An undesirable outcome can be anticipated if a therapist, who assumes that bottling up feelings is harmful and discharging them is beneficial encourages a patient to express anger. This approach interferes with finding out what is responsible for the anger and why expressing it is difficult. Also, the patient is placed in the position of a child who is told what to do. And finally, if the patient does express anger, perhaps of a petulant or temper tantrum type, he or she is likely to be enmeshed in additional (social) problems.

Comments indicating that the therapist sides with a patient and supports the patient's struggle with another person may have undesirable consequences. Such an outcome is to be expected if the therapist agrees with the patient and makes a statement such as "It seems that your wife (husband) does not understand you."

By using a spouse as an opponent, an internal struggle may be converted into an external battle. At best, internal conflicts, with the tension they engender, are difficult to abide, and at worst they are avoided at almost all cost. The conflicts may be of many sorts—how to discipline children (to be lenient or strict), how to spend money (to be frugal or extravagant), or what to do about weight gain (to diet or to continue overeating). These are only a few of the more common problems. Rather than deal with an intrapsychic conflict, for example, a husband may find it easier to place his wife on one side of an issue (usually on the side toward which she leans) and to do battle with her. Thereby internal tensions are reduced or even relieved. The cost to a marriage, however, may be considerable. Some marriages are able to withstand this type of wear and tear, especially if it is not constant; others are not. The task in psychotherapy is to make the person aware of how he or she is using a marital partner and to help him or her face the issue and deal with it more directly—not to take sides and help perpetuate the battle.

Summaries, Recapitulations, and Confrontations

A summary is the therapist's condensation of a thesis developed by the patient, and a recapitulation is the therapist's restatement of a thesis. Because summaries and recapitulations are similar and essentially serve the same purpose, they will be discussed together. Some therapists are reluctant to offer summaries or recapitulations because of concern that in doing so the obvious is stated or restated, thereby belittling the patient's good intelligence. There is this danger, but if well-timed, these interventions can be of appreciable value (Wolberg 1954).

Summaries and recapitulations sharpen the focus on a particular issue. Moreover, hearing another person say the very same thing that one has said may cast a new light on it. This experience is similar to that of rereading a book and suddenly discovering—as though for the first time—a facet hardly noticed previously. A summary or recapitulation may also be somewhat like a translation. If the patient states a matter in coldly intellectual terms, the therapist, by translating the message into a language highly charged with emotional overtones, may make it more meaningful.

Summaries and recapitulations, insofar as they are accurate, also serve to increase rapport. Hearing one's thoughts, feelings, and conflicts accurately summarized is a confirmation of the therapist's empathy.

Occasionally a recapitulation may take on the qualities of a confrontation. Devereux (1951) pointed to this when he stated,

> Confrontation . . . consists essentially in a rewording of the patient's own statements, especially in the form of "calling a spade a spade." Nothing is added to the patient's statement, nor is anything subtracted. . . . In simplest terms, confrontation is a

> device whereby the patient's attention is directed to the bare factual content of his actions or statements. . . .

Acknowledgments

In the treatment situation the therapist's responses are mainly questions, informative comments, and interpretations. Summaries, recapitulations, and confrontations are used but much less frequently. Still another infrequent but important response is acknowledgment of what Greenson (1972) referred to as "a good piece of insight on the patient's part."

Greenson introduced a word of caution, however, in affirming the importance of the patient's insight. He stated,

> Acknowledging that a patient has made a valuable insight often seduces the patient into attempting to make immediate interpretations of his own material. He becomes a "junior psychoanalyst," a caricature of a working alliance. This has to be demonstrated and interpreted so that the analysis does not deteriorate into an educational seminar or a guessing game. Tact is required because we do not want to crush the patient's healthy wish to do some of the analytic work himself.

Summary

Interpretations, comments, summaries, recapitulations, and confrontations are all active interventions by the therapist. Interpretations attempt to bring unconscious processes into conscious awareness and thus, by definition, play a major role in insight-oriented psychotherapy. Informative comments serve a variety of purposes—social, educational, and confrontational—while summaries and recapitulations help to maintain a therapeutic focus.

8

How Psychotherapy Works

The emphasis thus far has been on the part played by the therapist's relationship to the patient and the role of technique in contributing to the therapeutic process. Less attention has been focused on the part played by the patient and on the limitations of psychotherapy in its ability to effect change. An analogy to a computer might be drawn: Psychotherapy can help "reprogram" but it cannot change "hard wiring." Patients can learn to correct perceptual distortions and develop new patterns of behavior. Yet, they vary, at a constitutional level, in terms of their intelligence, their affectual reactivity, and even in their style of thinking. These conditions must be understood so that too much will not be promised and a sense of failure engendered by setting impossible goals.

Mental Set

In psychotherapy, the patient's mental set is of fundamental importance. By mental set is meant a prevailing state of mind that determines in considerable measure how a person, object, or event is viewed and what the reaction to it will be.

Mood influences mental set and, in a sense, can be regarded as one of its building blocks. Other components of mental set include the inclination toward optimism or pessimism, the tendency to take matters lightly or seriously, and the readiness to react with confidence or despair. These and many other qualities shape mental set. In recent years, medications such as antidepressants have provided therapists with the means to chemically alter mood and, through mood, attitude—at least to some extent.

Mental set is also related to temperament, which "like intelligence and physique might be said to designate a class of 'raw material' from which personality is fashioned" (Allport 1961). By temperament is meant the inborn type of reactivity, style as well as intensity of responsiveness. Temperament, like intelligence and physique, leans heavily on gene determination and is therefore the aspect of personality most dependent on heredity (Cloninger 1987). Allport (1961) added, "Temperament refers to the chemical climate or 'internal weather' in which personality evolves. The more anchored a disposition is in native constitutional soil the more likely it is to be spoken of as temperament."

Mental set is the product of genetic, constitutional, metabolic, and psychological forces. A particular biological makeup can be shaped or altered by biological events. Examples are depression resulting from reserpine or carcinoma of the pancreas and the relief of depression resulting from the withdrawal of antihypertensive medication or the prescription of antidepressant medication.

Although the importance of mental set has been recognized, the efforts to change it have been limited. More attention has been paid to the part played by attitude in marital therapy than in various types of individual therapy. This is not surprising in view of the fact that it is often glaringly evident that the attitude toward marital problems, more than the problems themselves, is the crucial consideration.

Determinants of Behavior

Psychic determinism, referring to the part played by unconscious forces in shaping behavior, is an important but probably overemphasized phenomenon. There are glaring examples of its operation. Clearly, it must be considered as the driving force when a woman marries four times and each husband, much to her surprise, turns out to be an alcoholic philanderer, similar in those respects to her father.

More often patterns of behavior are the product of complex forces including biology (genetics and endowment), fortuity (occurrences ascribed to chance), conditions beyond one's control (being sent to a concentration camp), and conscious deliberations and personal decisions.

Fortuity is almost surely the crucial factor when a person in a car stopped at a red light is rear-ended. To attempt to ascribe the accident and injury to psychic determinism would seem implausible and only serve to alienate a patient. Moreover, it would lead to unreasonable and unrealistic expectations of what might be accomplished by psychotherapy.

There are both biological circumstances and psychological trauma that result in states that are relatively refractory to psychotherapeutic interventions. Fortuity remains part of life, and the ability to deal with many of its effects may be crucial. With these caveats in mind, we will now turn to what psychotherapy can do and how the process works.

Therapeutic Mechanisms

Insight

Popular books, movies, and television productions have often and erroneously dramatized the remarkable removal of symptoms brought about by the recovery of a childhood memory and the interpretation of its unconscious meaning. Unfortunately, in real life such a dramatic scenario is extremely rare. Instead, there is the laborious task in which insight is a tool rather than an end product.

It may be discerned that a patient repeats a particular pattern of behavior over and over again in psychotherapy as well as elsewhere. The pattern may be gross and clearly visible or subtle and indistinct. In any event, once a pattern can be distinguished, the next step is to identify its unconscious determinants. In addressing this subject, Strupp (1972) stated,

> The "insights" which the patient gains . . . may be valuable in their own right; they may prove rewarding in demonstrating to the patient wishes, impulses and fantasies whose existence he only dimly suspected; they may be educational in a variety of other ways; however they do not change behavior.

The issue of change was also addressed in the following terms:

> The process of psychotherapy is designed not to impose change on the patient but to create conditions within the context of the therapeutic relationship which will allow changes to occur within the patient. (Waterhouse and Strupp 1984)

Although insight does not in itself bring about change, it may prepare the way for or facilitate change. By becoming aware of a pattern of behavior, the patient may have an option that did not exist before. It may be possible to get out of a rut that has been dug deeper and deeper through the years and attempt to open a new path.

A fundamental objective of insight-oriented psychotherapy is to increase self-knowledge. Classically this is accomplished by making the unconscious conscious. As previously stated, usually the most meaningful learning occurs in the transference. To find the old blueprint that shapes present-day behavior, it is not necessary to induce regression; present-day behavior will reveal the blueprint, usually unconscious, that shaped it.

The following case note is an example of a repetitive pattern that came to light in psychotherapy.

> *A 35-year-old woman went from one heterosexual relationship to another, none lasting longer than one year and all of them remaining somewhat shallow. It soon became evident that she could not bear to be alone and yet she feared closeness. In psychotherapy she became aware of a repetitive pattern of attachment and retreat that previously had been responsible for her multiple brief liaisons, which included three marriages. A further step would be for the patient to learn about the unconscious roots of her pattern of behavior.*

In the following case note, the "pieces" were assembled by the therapist to form a pattern that the patient could recognize and act on.

> *An attractive 35-year-old woman sought psychiatric treatment because she felt guilty about her sexual behavior. Early in her marriage of 10 years she had had thoughts about having extramarital affairs but had not acted on her fantasy until recently. She explained that she had had very little premarital experience and now she wanted to have the chance to experiment before she was too old. Also, she was bored and depressed, and her escapades added some "sparkle" to her life.*
>
> *Six months before, the patient had had a hysterectomy. When asked what effect the operation had on her picture of her desirability as a woman, she said "I don't know. There is just something gone." When asked if she felt less like a woman, she said, "Well, I don't know unless I have been trying to prove I'm not." It was pointed out that her need to prove that she was still desirable as a woman led to the behavior that caused her guilt. She responded, "I see it. . . . I see what you are talking about."*

In this instance the patient provided the pieces and the therapist put them together, making them form a clear picture. Two events—the multiple sexual encounters and the hysterectomy—had not been connected by the patient until the therapist pointed out the effect the operation had had on her self-image. Once aware of the nature of her struggle, she was able to discontinue the behavior that she recognized could be destructive.

Interpretations and the Transference

The most distinctive feature of insight-oriented psychotherapy is the interpretation that imparts information to patients about their unconscious processes. There are several ways in which the nature of these processes can be inferred. One of the most common is recognizing that a statement *by analogy* refers to feelings that are difficult to express directly. For example, in speaking about a person who did not hear something important because he was inattentive, it could be inferred that the patient was speaking about the therapist.

The transference is likely to provide the clearest picture of unconscious processes at work. For example, a patient mentioned that for some reason she did not understand why she had the notion that her previous hour, which had been canceled, had been given to someone else. Following this, she spoke of how wonderful the therapist was, making one saccharine-coated remark after another. In the therapeutic encounter, she behaved as she did in her everyday life; she was sweet to the therapist (parent), who she believed preferred someone else (sibling) to her. In dealing with the situation, the pseudo-sweetness was pointed out first. Its connection with angry or hurt feelings in response to a fantasied rebuff was then interpreted. Finally, its roots in earlier experiences were unearthed. This approach is consistent with psychoanalytic practice in which the defense is interpreted first, then what is defended against, and finally the genetic basis of the reaction. Learning of this sort, which is emotionally experienced, may open the way to a change in the pattern of the patient's behavior.

Corrective Emotional Experience

A Corrective emotional experience occurs when patients are reexposed, under favorable circumstances, to emotional situations which they could not handle in the past.

> Because the therapist's attitude is different from that of the authoritative person of the past, he gives the patient an opportunity to face again and again, under more favorable circum-

> stances, those emotional situations which were formerly unbearable and to deal with them in a manner different from the old. (Alexander and French 1946)

To bring about a corrective emotional experience, therapists' attitudes need not be contrived; their usual stance should create the desired situation.

Deconditioning

Deconditioning occurs in most types of psychotherapy, and even psychoanalysis is not an exception. Patients, whether sitting up or lying on a couch, feel protected by the therapist, a parent substitute, and in that situation may be able gradually to face certain issues that otherwise would be avoided. They do so by essentially creating their own hierarchy and progressively tackling more and more frightening subjects.

A patient, feeling supported and protected by a therapist, may become brave enough to try a new type of relating (for example, dating). With success, there may be a ripple effect consisting of generally improved social behavior. A favorable reaction evoked by the new behavior will in turn reinforce it, thus setting off a beneficial cycle.

For patients who usually act first and think later, psychotherapy is a new kind of learning experience. Not only is the process reflective and introspective, but whenever possible the therapist, alert to small clues, points out what the patient is poised to do. Thus, an inclination or an impulse is scrutinized when it is first taking shape and before it has resulted in action. The effect is to decondition one mode of conduct (to act first) and to condition another (to think first). Of course, the question at the onset of psychotherapy is "Will the patient be able to tolerate thoughtful deliberation and delay?"

Borrowing the Therapist's Ego/Superego

During and after psychotherapy patients often view life events, thoughts, and feelings in terms of how they imagine their therapist might respond. This phenomenon is similar to that encountered in the child or adolescent as a part of the learning process.

A patient confronted by a certain situation might wonder, "What would Dr. X think or say?" The patient then looks at the situation through Dr. X's "glasses" and as a result may be less self-critical or less prone to act impulsively. Gradually, the qualities borrowed from the therapist may be incorporated and experienced as a part of oneself.

This therapeutic mechanism of borrowing a part of the therapist is concretely demonstrated by the following clinical vignette, which was reported previously (Hollender 1959).

> *A young woman with bodily complaints and ideas of reference was initially seen on a weekly basis. After a few months her appointments were "spaced and spanned" until she was seen only when she called to request an appointment.*
>
> *Ideas of reference, which had ceased soon after treatment began, recurred two years later when she attended a ceremony for one of her sisters, who was becoming a nun. She explained that the ceremony brought her back under the sway of her stern, almost unbearable, conscience. It was not enough then for her to remind herself of how her therapist would view matters. She had to see him to combat the resurgence of her oppressive superego. As she explained, "I needed a refill."*

In this instance the therapist was adopted as a surrogate parent, and his attitude was taken over. His standard, however, was in a sense like a foreign body; it was ingested but did not really become part of the patient. Hence, from time to time she had to remind herself of how he would react. Usually a mental image was adequate, but sometimes his physical presence was required.

The Statement of an Authority

The statements of the therapist as an expert on human behavior and feelings may have a salutary effect. The following are two examples.

> *A young woman stated that she believed she felt better because of a statement the therapist made during the previous hour. The statement was that she could not expect to function up to par when she was depressed. Somehow that had relieved her greatly, but she was not sure why. When the therapist commented that sometimes people become depressed about being depressed, she agreed and then explained that, being raised as a member of a fundamentalist religion, she was told she was supposed to be happy. If she woke up feeling glum, she would say her*

prayers and hope that she would soon feel better. It was pointed out that when depressed and functioning poorly she felt bad or sinful. She responded that she even felt like a sinner when she was sick, especially if she was irritable.

The therapist's comments were really nothing more than generalizations, and hardly more than stating the obvious, but in this instance they evoked an unanticipated response. They gave the patient permission to feel depressed without feeling guilty. Of course, it was not the statements alone; it was that the statements were backed by "medical authority." The interchange with the therapist served to make the patient aware of an attitude and its source. Because there was no binding emotional force involved, it was possible to revise or update the attitude.

Another patient, upon returning from a trip, felt extremely upset when her little son kept a distance from her and told her to go away. She often thought of herself as a bad mother and consequently she reacted strongly to her son's behavior. In this situation the therapist pointed out that the reaction the patient encountered was common and that it was often upsetting to parents, especially if they misinterpreted it. Because of the child's attachment to her, he resented it when she left him and was paying her back by keeping a distance from her and saying, "Go away. I don't need you. Because you rejected me, I will get back at you by rejecting you."

When therapists provide some perspective, they are assuming the role of an expert in human behavior—which they are.

Handling Unacceptable Feelings

The suppression and repression of anger may be of etiological significance for phobias or for physical symptoms such as headaches and anxiety with hyperventilation. In such instances the objective is not to encourage patients to spew out their anger, which sometimes takes the form of temper tantrums or "blind" rage. Therapists who encourage nondiscriminant expression of emotions may find a paradoxical effect to such behavior: the nondirected anger causes complications that reinforce the patients' resolve to remain emotionally constricted. Rather, the objective is to help patients see connections between unexpressed feelings and physical reactions and then to learn how to address anger-producing situations before the feelings become explosive.

These patients usually have to come to realize, too, that a wish is not the same as a deed—that their wishes, even death wishes, do not kill.

Symptom Removal

In medical practice, symptom removal as the sole aim of treatment is often frowned on. To suppress the cough of a patient with pulmonary tuberculosis would be little more than palliative; the destructive process would go on unabated until a downhill course ended in death. To remove a symptom caused by a psychiatric disorder—for example, a phobia—is often quite a different matter. In this instance the outside world might be opened up for a person who had been housebound. Once out of the house, the patient might return to work and renew social ties with relatives and friends. The result would be an upward spiral; whether the cause of the symptom—in this instance, the phobia—was discovered or not is of no concern.

The Therapist and Learning

The part played by the patient's relationship to the therapist has already been noted in this and other chapters of the book. Still, some additional comments will be made about this important learning process.

The life experience provided by the therapist creates an impact on the patient in several ways. For example, as a result of being treated with respect—in that thoughts, beliefs, and behavior are taken seriously and not disparaged—the patient may undergo a change in attitude or self-concept. Although the change may not be radical, it may be sufficient to induce some alteration in behavior toward other people, who in turn may respond more positively and perhaps set an upward spiral in motion.

Another example of learning in the relationship involves self-expression. A patient who is afraid of being aggressive might first become mildly assertive in dealing with the therapist. Little by little, such expression might become more open. In this instance, as in many others, the experience would complement learning acquired through interpretations and other interventions. It stands in relationship to interpretations like an illustration in a book to the printed text. (This type of experience should not be confused with one in which the patient is encouraged to express himself or herself as a form of catharsis.)

An admired teacher is often emulated; similarly, a therapist may serve as the model for a patient. This kind of influence leads to imitation, identification, and learning by example. For some patients it is an unavoidable consequence of the therapeutic situation; for others it may be fostered. An ideal culture medium for its growth is provided by marked regression and the imposition of demands for conformity in a needful person who can ill afford to alienate anyone upon whom he or she is dependent.

The impact of the therapist's attitude is illustrated by the following vignette.

> *A woman often reacted to everyday situations as though they were major crises. The therapist, regarding the situations as though they were no more eventful than the usual changes in the weather, conveyed an attitude of forbearance and detachment. After a while, but before learning why she reacted so dramatically, the patient began to describe events in a less emotional and more matter of fact manner. She seemed to have taken on the therapist's attitude, or perhaps she had learned by example.*

A similar influence may be exerted by one friend on another. Some changes brought about in this way are ephemeral, but others may be long lasting.

Unorthodox Tactics (The Argyrol Phenomenon)

Otolaryngologists speak out against the use of Argyrol (silver vitelline) in the nose, pointing out that its supposed anti-infective effect is nonphysiologic or even antiphysiologic. And yet these same practitioners may keep a small bottle of Argyrol in their office. When asked why they do, they explain that now and again, perhaps once or twice a year or even less often, they encounter a patient who benefits from the judicious use of Argyrol and is unresponsive to more physiologic and conventional approaches. They would not speak in favor of using Argyrol or write about it, however, because of their concern that it might be used promiscuously and hence abused. Its potential for harm would worry them if it were in general use.

Probably every specialty of medicine has its Argyrol phenomenon. Certainly some psychiatrists keep the psychiatric equivalent of Argyrol carefully tucked away in their offices, an unorthodox approach they may choose to follow occasionally to cope with a specific situation, an approach that they might justify but not one they would recommend to others for general use.

Greenbaum (1986) presented the following vignette that illustrates the "Argyrol phenomenon."

> *A single woman in her mid-30s came for treatment after being caught shoplifting. The manager of the department store did not call the police, but he advised her to seek psychiatric help. At eight years of age, in a brief period, the patient lost both parents to tuberculosis. She was sent to an orphanage where she remained for the next six years. Because of the scarcity of food, the children were forced to steal. When she was transferred to a foster home, the foster mother told her that the agency did not pay enough money to provide such extras as fruit, candies, or attractive clothing, and to obtain them she would have to steal. And this she did.*
>
> *After three years of psychotherapy, the patient had made great strides in many areas, but not in regard to shoplifting. One day after she reported a new theft, the therapist decided to abandon his usual stance, and he reprimanded her severely, the way a caring parent would. She was devastated, but the punishment worked. The fear of losing her therapist's acceptance and respect caused her to give up the learned antisocial behavior.*

Summing Up

The relationship provided by the therapist exerts a significant effect in several ways. The hope of obtaining relief from distress or of obtaining help in resolving problems is likely to have a positive effect at the outset. As a result of feeling bolstered or supported, the patient may reach out to others or take some form of positive action. If the response evoked is favorable, additional steps may be taken and an upward spiral created.

The therapist, as a role model, may serve as an object for imitation and identification. The nature of the therapeutic situation is likely to be such that it provides for a corrective experience, and it does so without contrivance. Moreover, patients may "borrow" what they picture as their therapist's more tolerant and flexible superego and use it in place of their own.

In terms of technique, insight gained by the patient with the help of interpretations does not in itself produce change. It does, however, prepare the way for change, and like education generally, it increases the options available.

As should be evident, therapy works in many ways, sometimes by direct action, other times as a catalyst, and still other times by preparing the way for change. And it should not be overlooked that occasionally the part played by external circumstances may be of considerable significance.

Psychotherapy Research

It has only been since World War II that systematic and concerted attempts have been made to assess the changes in patients over time and to link the changes to particular therapeutic operations. The difficulties in such research have been many and great, and consequently progress has been small and slow. Still the effort continues to be made. Strupp et al. (1977) insist that "there must be some way of documenting the occurrence of change, difficult and fallible as such demonstrations may turn out to be."

In recent years an increasing number of centers have become involved in psychotherapy research, and their focus has been on both process and outcome. One professional organization, The Society of Psychotherapy Research, is entirely devoted to this subject. Some research has been initiated by a perceived need to demonstrate cost-effectiveness in order to maintain the legitimacy of reimbursement by third-party payers. Other questions addressed include the following:

- What type of psychotherapy is effective for what kind of problem?
- What type of psychotherapy is effective for what kind of patient?
- What is the appropriate length of treatment?
- Are the effects of psychotherapy transient or enduring?

Summary

Patients' mental set may exert a substantial influence on how they respond to psychotherapy. Moreover, it will have much to do with receptivity to learning or the lack of it.

In considering how psychotherapy works there are those changes attributable to the special relationship provided by therapists and those attributable to their technique. Both play a part in various ways in dynamic forms of psychotherapy. In insight-oriented psychotherapy, in which the emphasis is on uncovering and interpreting unconscious processes, the focus is on the part played by technique. In supportive psychotherapy, in which the emphasis is on bolstering defenses, the focus is on the part played by the relationship to the therapist. It should be understood, however, that in almost all instances in which psychotherapy works, both factors are involved.

9

Guidelines and Stratification

There are no clearly drawn maps to direct the therapist after the opening moves in therapy, but there are general guidelines suggesting which routes to take. These guidelines, in conjunction with the principle of stratification, should prove helpful.

Guidelines

When the therapist comes to a fork in the road where an intervention in the form of a question, comment, or interpretation would be in order, the following guidelines should help the therapist decide which branch of the road to take. This list, of course, is not meant to be exhaustive, and other experienced psychotherapists could no doubt suggest additions. Our guidelines are as follows:

Focus on the here-and-now rather than the past. The following case note is illustrative:

> *A 62-year-old woman, in psychotherapy for four months, began her weekly hour by launching into a description of her early married life. While her husband attended a fine Eastern graduate school, they traveled in a select social circle. In relating this information, she indulged in much name dropping. Recently, following a liver biopsy that revealed cirrhosis, she had admitted to being a closet alcoholic who drank much more than the glass of wine a day she had previously acknowledged.*
>
> *The therapist wondered what he should do in dealing with old historical material. Should he make an interpretation? Or should he let it pass without comment? Actually the crucial issue was in the present, not the past, and it was specifically that the drinking problem, which the*

> *patient had tried to hide, made her feel ashamed. To dampen or counterbalance this narcissistic blow, she turned (or returned) to a time when she felt important. She was telling her therapist (and herself) to remember that she was once a person of substance. To this the therapist might have commented that she reacted to the revelation of alcoholism as a blow to her self-esteem. Doing so would have given her the opportunity to express and discuss her feelings.*

To take appropriate action the therapist needed first to ask, "Why did the patient suddenly begin to talk about the past?" In previous meetings, she had focused on present-day problems. The missing piece was the revelation of her drinking behavior and what it meant to acknowledge that she was an alcoholic. With this information, her communication became clear: The patient made a narcissistic move to counteract a narcissistic blow. In effect she stated, "I may not be much now, but I was once somebody important."

Transference and other characteristics of the therapist-patient relationship are of prime importance. This guideline is actually a corollary of the previous one because the therapeutic relationship exists in the here-and-now. There are two major reasons for focusing on the therapeutic relationship. First, "learning" within this context is much more vivid, more emotionally charged, and therefore more telling. Second, until problems in the therapist-patient relationship are dealt with, it may be difficult to address other areas of conflict.

In working with dreams (particularly a long dream), the focus initially should be on the portion that seems to relate to the therapist-patient relationship (see Chapter 10).

The "presenting part" should be "delivered" first. In psychotherapy, grief usually must be dealt with before other issues will surface. For example, a woman being seen once a week in psychotherapy was told by her man friend that he would not marry her. She was very upset, almost distraught. Under the circumstances, what is the therapist's immediate task? It is to provide the patient with an opportunity to talk about her feelings, to listen attentively to her, and perhaps to make some comment about how difficult or disheartening the situation is for her. It is not likely to be a time for interpretations; the work of therapy should not be pushed when the patient needs a chance to grieve. Clichés intended to be consoling, such as "It's still not too late to find someone else," "Time will take care of things," or "Things could be worse" are horribly inappropriate.

Later in the same hour the same patient recounted a dream in which one tooth after another was falling out of her mouth. In associating to the dream, she mentioned her concern about growing old. It was then suggested that she seemed afraid that she might become too old before finding a mate. This opened an important area for reflection and discussion.

Focus on the meta communication before dealing with the content. When a patient wallows in self-pity, it is pointless to talk about an insensitive remark made by a friend or about the complaints leveled at a spouse. The frame of mind colors everything—a dark color. Until the self-pity is brought into focus, discussed, and lifted, everything will be just another miserable experience.

With dreams, as with other statements, the meta communication (the context) should be dealt with before the content. For example if a patient who rarely reported dreams suddenly flooded the hours with pages of written out dreams, this phenomenon and not the content should be first addressed.

First ascertain if the patient's assumption is warranted. A college student expressed great concern about a small lump behind his ear. He feared that his ear might have to be amputated. (This reaction occurred during psychotherapy when he was preoccupied with castration fear.) The first step was to point out to the patient that he made a big leap from a small lump to the amputation of an ear. How did he explain this leap? It was necessary to establish the fact that his assumption was not warranted by the circumstances before looking for its unconscious roots.

Therapists should not assume that patients share their outlook. It may seem that a patient wishes to change a character trait that causes him or her or others to feel uncomfortable. But this is often far from the case. For instance, a perfectionist who grumbles about the burden created by perfectionism may covertly place a high value on it and would be extremely reluctant to entertain the possibility of relinquishing it. The starting point, therefore, is a discussion of the desire to hold on to the perfectionism. The patient must be made aware that a virtue has been made out of what perhaps was once a necessity. If the therapist assumes that there is a strong wish to relinquish the perfectionism and proceeds on that basis, the effort is probably doomed to fail.

Look for the real issue. In the following instance a narcissistic problem masqueraded as a sexual problem. For the patient to have a learning experience under the circumstance, the therapist would have to point out the real issue and keep the focus on it.

> *A young man whose behavior seemed to express the need to be "one up" complained about his wife's muted response to sex. She had only small, controlled orgasms instead of large, wild ones, and this infuriated him. He felt sure she had a problem and wondered if behavior therapy would be recommended for it.*

The patient was obviously basically concerned about his own manliness. To him, his wife's reaction meant either that he was inadequate or she was inhibited. If he could assume it was the latter, he would succeed in warding off a narcissistic blow.

The therapist, in this instance, focused on the wrong issue. Based on a preconception about sexual dysfunction, he commented that sexual difficulties in marriage usually mean that both partners have problems. In all likelihood the patient understood this to mean, "It's not just your wife; you, too, have problems. You are inadequate." The patient responded with an outburst in which he depreciated the therapist and clearly tried to put him down.

In this instance, a narcissistic struggle took place in a sexual arena. The therapist should have asked why the patient had the need to use his wife's reaction to sex as a measure of his manliness or adequacy. By so doing the unrewarding interchange between therapist and patient might have been averted.

The following case note is of another instance in which focusing on the right issue is crucial.

> *A 27-year-old single woman, who had presented to the clinic with the chief complaint of confusion over her sexual identity, was seen in psychotherapy once a week. In the fifth session, she stated, "I feel more comfortable with you when I'm wearing a dress [rather than slacks]."*

Therapist: *Why is that?*
Patient: *Because I think you think dresses are more feminine.*
Therapist: *I do?*
Patient: *Not you as a doctor, but you as a man.*
Therapist: *Do you mean all men?*

Patient: *Yes.*
Therapist: *Why?*
Patient: *Because women wear dresses.*
Therapist: *But today they wear pants, too.*
Patient: *I know, but . . . mother told me ladies dress up and don't wear jeans. . . . Jack came over the other night and I was wearing jeans and a T-shirt. . . . I really felt uncomfortable.*
Therapist: *Why?*
Patient: *I just didn't feel feminine. . . . I guess I think pants make me look "dykey."*

The important consideration was that the patient wanted to look feminine in the eyes of her therapist rather than whether or not slacks were feminine. The questions the therapist asked led down the wrong road.

Here is another example in which focusing on the real issue was crucial.

A young woman engaged in psychiatric treatment as a precondition for readmission to the top-flight college from which she had been suspended. She was also required to take courses at a college of her choice for one year and perform well. During 10 interviews she had been encouraged to bring some order into her chaotic and tumultuous everyday life, and she had made considerable strides in doing so. At the 11th interview, she was dressed up. She explained that she had dressed up to make a good appearance so she could obtain a small bank loan to pay her tuition. She was given the loan even though technically she failed to qualify for it. She then explained that when she dressed up she was not her real self.

At this point the therapist might have suggested to the patient that the dressed-up young woman *was* a part of herself. Instead he asked, "What is your real self?" thereby, in effect, concurring with her point. The patient responded that she did not know what her real self was, but when she wore good clothes she knew she was a phony. She connected this with living with a family she described as insincere and in which a certain type of conduct and dress was required. Perhaps, she suggested, she was reacting against dressing up now because of her past experiences.

Too often, the assumption is made that there is a real and an unreal self rather than that there are several real selves or, more precisely, several facets of the real self. There is the real self that is owned (acknowledged) and there is the real self that is disowned (denied).

If the therapist accepts being dressed up as phony, then the issue is "Why can't you be real?" If, on the other hand, the therapist maintains that being dressed up is real but disowned, then the issue is "Why is the behavior disowned?"

Adult behavior should be favored when the focus can be on it or on childlike behavior. A young man told his therapist that his mother encouraged him to consume large helpings of food that she prepared for him and then berated him for being overweight. Should the therapist explore why the patient's mother treats him like a child? Or should the therapist ask the patient how he handles the situation? The first approach assumes the patient might be a poor, helpless child, the second that he is an adult capable of making choices.

Do not automatically accept the patients' assumptions as valid. There are times when their assumptions should be challenged. How should a therapist respond to a patient who states, "I cannot make her [his wife] happy, and this is terribly upsetting"? Should the therapist inquire why he cannot make her happy? Or should the question be posed, "Is it really your responsibility to make her happy?" This example highlights the importance of scrutinizing premises. It is easy—and tempting—to accept the patient's assumption that he should make his wife happy, but if that were the case he would be left with a huge burden. It is one thing to contribute to the happiness of another person, but quite another to be held responsible for it.

A person may feel justified in expecting a partner to know what is needed or desired and to provide it without being asked. To have to ask, so it is maintained, ruins everything. Actually, the person is behaving like a preverbal infant whose mother might be expected to fathom what is needed or desired. The assumption that a partner should know what to supply without being asked is open to question. (See also our discussion of "real self" or "disowned part of oneself," earlier in this chapter within the section entitled "Look for the real issue").

What cannot be expressed directly may be voiced in an analogy selected unconsciously. A striking example follows.

A therapist informed a patient whom he had seen for only four appointments that he thought she had progressed so well that her treatment could be terminated. She acknowledged she was indeed doing very well and agreed that treatment could be terminated. A few minutes later, however, she mentioned that a teacher had skipped her daughter one grade in school, and she went on to comment, with considerable feeling, that she did not approve of teachers who pushed children ahead too rapidly—the therapist heard the message.

The following case note is another instance in which a message was sent in the form of an analogy.

A young man debated about mowing the lawn but finally decided to mow it. He said, "So I go out there and start the mower up, and I am halfway done and I ride over a nest of yellow jackets. Do you know how angry they get—about a dozen stings worth all over my legs and arms." The patient mentioned that the summer was half gone and while others had been dating, he was just sitting around. The therapist suggested that perhaps he had not dated because he was afraid of stirring up a nest of yellow jackets. He responded that sitting around doing nothing was getting to him. The therapist commented that the patient found sitting around dull but he was afraid of what he might run into if he dated.

The practical approach should be favored over the analytic. It would be expecting too much to assume that therapists will avoid all expressions of bias. And from a practical standpoint it might even be undesirable for them to do so. The following are two clinical examples in which a practical approach was favored.

A 29-year-old woman, short and obese, had never been out on a date. The first dream she reported in psychotherapy was of a flowered wallpaper, an apt description of herself—the wallflower. After approximately 10 months in treatment she began to struggle with feelings about her therapist that she found difficult to acknowledge or accept. At that time she began to date. Although there was much to suggest that she did so because she was eager to live out her feelings with her dates rather than face her feelings about her therapist, it would have been unthinkable to interpret the acting out. Her behavior had such potential for positive learning that the therapist felt that nothing should be done to disturb it. His stance was practical rather than analytic.

Another patient, a 37-year-old woman who repetitively backed away from relationships with men at a point of closeness, was beginning to put distance between herself and her 18-year-old live-in boyfriend. She was repeating an old pattern.

Was this the time and circumstance for the therapist to point out what she did repetitively, or was her present relationship so unbalanced that nothing should be said that would interfere with its dissolution? The situation was dealt with as a practical rather than an analytic issue and nothing was said.

In the two examples cited above, bias, based on a value system, influenced the therapist's approach. In these instances the situation appeared so clear and compelling that the course to follow seemed self-evident. Accordingly, a practical approach prevailed over an analytic one. The parameters created, however, probably should be addressed later.

The approach we have suggested here is not without danger. Anytime the nature of a psychotherapeutic intervention is strongly influenced by the therapist's value system, there is the danger that the patient's self-determination will be submerged. The two examples cited are relatively benign and noncontroversial. But what if they had involved religion, abortion, birth control, or similar issues?

Stratification

In psychotherapy, levels of reaction may be identified by the therapist and pointed out to the patient. The following clinical note illustrates this phenomenon.

Mrs. D, who is 21 years old, married for four years, and the mother of a two-year-old son, was overpowered by two men who assaulted and raped her when her car broke down on a dark country road. Since then her relationship with her husband had been strained, and she tended to be irritable and impatient with her son. She had become wary and suspicious: she would not sit in a chair with her back to the door, and she sometimes wondered if people were talking

> *about her. Nightmares were frequent and in them she would thrash about and scream. Mrs. D and her husband had both been brought up to believe that a person should have sexual intercourse only with one's spouse. It therefore disturbed them that Mrs. D had had sexual intercourse with two other men even if it was against her will.*
>
> *In spite of the circumstances of the rape, Mrs. D wondered if she had done something to provoke sexually aggressive behavior in the two men. As far as she knew, she had never seen them before, but still she entertained the possibility that they might have seen her at a night spot where she often went dancing with her husband. She felt troubled and guilty.*
>
> *According to Mrs. D, her husband was not a jealous man but he would usually ask what detained her if she was late returning home. Prior to the time she was assaulted and raped, she simply replied briefly and that sufficed. More recently she refused to answer him, and this created friction. The therapist commented that she pointed a finger at herself in spite of the fact that she knew she had done nothing to provoke the rape. Then, being in this self-accusatory frame of mind, she reacted to her husband's question as an accusation and became defensive. She stated that she had not considered this possibility, but she was aware that her reaction resulted in undesirable repercussions.*

Mrs. D expressed a desire to talk abut her experience and to alter the pattern stemming from it. The feelings that she recognized were fear at the time of the assault, then anger and rage at her assailants, and more recently guilt. The following stratification could be delineated:

On a superficial level,

- Mrs. D feels guilty—"Did I do something to provoke the assault and rape?"
- Because of her guilty frame of mind, she reacts to her husband's question (about why she was late) as an accusation and becomes defensive.
- The result is marital friction.
- The connection between her guilt and her reaction to her husband's question was not recognized until it was pointed out.
- The interpretation should relieve some marital friction, but it is not likely to relieve her guilt.

At a deeper level,

- Mrs. D's guilt, which she perceives as at least somewhat unreasonable, in all likelihood stems from a repressed (or unconscious) rape fantasy.
- Rape fantasies are common and in childhood serve to reduce or disown responsibility for forbidden sexual wishes.
- To be relieved of guilt, Mrs. D must become aware that the guilt largely stems from a childhood fantasy.

Therapy consists mainly of making the patient aware of connections she failed to perceive on her own. The first connection was between the question her husband asked ("Why were you detained?") and her reaction to the question as though she was being incriminated. Prior to the rape she had not reacted in this manner. If she could now see the question as relatively innocuous, some tension would be relieved.

The second connection was between the recent event (the rape) and her childhood fantasy (rape fantasy). Because this common fantasy was reactivated by her experience, she reacted with guilt, as though her wish was responsible for what happened to her.

Once the patient recognizes the connections, especially if she does so with strong affect, she is likely to experience some relief.

The concept (and therapeutic principle) of stratification is that psychological situations may have multiple levels of meaning and therefore different levels of interpretation. It is desirable to deal with the most superficial issues first and then, similar to peeling layers of an onion, address progressively deeper issues. It would have been inappropriate, and therapeutically counterproductive, for the therapist in the above case note to have started therapy by interpreting the woman's rape fantasies.

Summary

As would be expected, clinical experience amply supports the contention that the most pressing and immediate problems should be addressed first. Problems in the here-and-now and particularly in the therapeutic relationship are of prime importance and must be continuously monitored and their meaning interpreted to the patient. The therapist needs to be on the lookout for decoys and reactions expressed in analogies or metaphors. When there is a choice, the focus should be on adult behavior rather than on regressive behavior.

10

Technical Considerations: Dream Interpretation, Resistance, and Regression

Some of the technical aspects of dynamic psychotherapy have already been considered. No discussion would be complete, however, without special attention being devoted to dream interpretation, resistance, and regression.

Dreams

Freud (1900) referred to dreams as "the royal road to the unconscious," and his book *The Interpretation of Dreams* was his magnum opus. Succeeding generations of therapists have been fascinated by dreams, much as Freud was, and have sought to understand the messages they contain. Although recent research has suggested that dreams may be important for the storage of memory and perhaps other aspects of brain function, it is the interpretation of dreams that is the primary concern of the psychotherapist.

The Nature of Dreams

From the standpoint of therapeutic value (as opposed to their possible physiological role), dreams can best be conceptualized by an analogy to modern art. The usual rules of time and space are suspended and, similar to a cubist painting, multiple, often contradictory facets may coexist. Because dreaming is a projective phenomenon, aspects of the dreamer may be represented by different persons. There may be a condensation of time, and the dreamer may simultaneously be an adult and a child, and important persons (or their symbolic representations) from different times in a patient's life may coexist in the dream. Thus, there is a fluidity of time and space. (Readers of Gabriel Garcia Marquez's novel *One Hundred Years of Solitude* will appreciate the similar lack of boundaries in that artistic work, in that the reader has difficulty determining whether the setting is in the past, present, or future.)

The dream provides a projective mechanism that may simultaneously have multiple meanings and potential for differing levels of interpretation. This concept of differing levels of meaning is also reflective of the principles of stratification presented in Chapter 9.

Contrary to the claims of popular paperback books sold in supermarkets, there are no universal symbolic meanings represented in dreams. The symbolism portrayed for any dreamer is reflective of that individual's life experiences and personal psychodynamics. At times, however, a dreamer will use some fairly consistent symbolism in his or her own dreams. For example, one young man had repetitive dreams about his automobile. It was apparent (and confirmed repetitively through associative material) that the automobile was a symbolic representation of his body. Although no hard and fast rule can be made, dreams of movement may reflect a patient's perception of the progress of therapy. As a general rule, the therapist should look first for those aspects of a dream that reflect upon what is happening in the here-and-now. Special attention should be paid to the possibility that a dream is a way the patient communicates feelings toward the therapist.

The Use of Dreams in Therapy

From what has been said, it should follow that dreams can facilitate the process of psychotherapy, and they can be used in forms of psychotherapy other than those that are insight-oriented.

Dreams can serve diagnostically to reflect affective states (for example, morbid themes may reflect depression, and frightening dreams may reflect anxiety). Dreams may also be used to elicit more information that is consciously available to the patient but has not previously been reported (e.g., suppressed, or thought to be irrelevant by the patient). Dreams can also be used to discern basic psychodynamic themes and the nature of the therapeutic relationship.

Some therapists routinely inquire about dreams during the evaluation period and explain that reporting dreams is often a helpful technique for gaining further insight. Other therapists avoid singling out dreams for special consideration, preferring to let the patient's selection of topics be spontaneous. During therapy, some therapists occasionally ask if patients remember recent dreams, but as a rule patients should be allowed to report dreams at their own instigation.

Technical Aspects of Dream Interpretation

Not all patients recall their dreams to the same extent, and these differences may reflect some physiological as well as psychological variations among individuals. For example, the capacity to remember dreams is not a characteristic of alexithymic individuals (Krystal 1979). Also, it is a paradoxical finding that a patient who reports many dreams may be using this behavior as a form of resistance in psychotherapy in order to avoid discussion of real-life problems.

The task of interpreting a dream is similar to understanding a poem. The focus should be on allusions or figurative references and on discerning what they mean to the patient, not on deep or so-called universal symbols. Also, the focus should be on the problem in the here-and-now, not on an underlying childhood struggle. As might be expected, the current situation will rekindle memories of old experiences so that it is possible to gain some understanding of the past from the dream. The task, however, is to begin with the present, which is the cathected layer. Later the present can be linked to the past.

To unravel the pictorial representations, it is usually necessary to obtain the thoughts or associations of the dreamer. Some therapists ask the patient to speak of whatever comes to mind when thinking of the dream, whereas others ask the patient to concentrate on or reflect about a specific portion of the dream. Still others merely listen as the patient continues to speak. Even if no associations are requested and no direct or explicit connections are forthcoming, it is a good working assumption that statements preceding and following the dream are related to it.

Some patients repeatedly wait until only a few minutes remain in the hour before relating a dream. One reason for doing so is the wish to prolong the session. Sensing or knowing the therapist's special interest in dreams, patients may use them in an effort to extend the hour beyond the regularly allotted time. When this pattern is recognized, the purpose for which the dream is used rather than its content should be the object of scrutiny.

Patients who are reluctant to face certain issues that seem to come to the fore in their dreams may also wait until the last few minutes to relate them. They appease their conscience by relating the dreams, but they avoid the crucial issues by running out of time before they can be addressed. In these instances the content of the dream should be scrutinized, but the reluctance to deal with the content must be dealt with first.

Only in unusual circumstances should patients be asked at the outset to talk about the meaning of a dream. The meaning should emerge based on associations and perhaps other connections that are made in discussing the dream. It must be kept in mind that the meaning of any particular dream must be set in the context of both the psychodynamic and current life circumstances of the dreamer (the "day residue"). As with other communications, it is important to discover the event that touched off the problem that is dealt with in the dream. Not only is it helpful in unraveling the meaning of the dream, but it often provides a logical lead-in to an interpretation.

Although, in a sense, dreams use a special code form, they can be decoded much as other communications are decoded. And as with other disguised messages, the interpretation that is offered is based on an understanding of the unconscious conflict.

Associations to the dream. The dream may serve to bring forth new ideas and/or different ways of looking at older information. The following dream was reported by a patient in the initial phases of insight-oriented psychotherapy.

> *"I was in the airport parking structure at Chicago looking for my car. I finally found it. It was a sleek, expensive European sports car but the wheels were missing." When asked for associations to the dream, the patient initially said he had none. But then, he remembered that he had been to Chicago recently on a job interview. He had been offered a position with an increase in prestige and pay but had refused it because of his wife's unwillingness to leave their home in a small Southern city. This bit of previously unreported information served to highlight several ongoing marital conflicts which previously had been suppressed. Because it was early in therapy, the therapist chose not to interpret the dream further, although the symbolism of the car without wheels suggested that the patient was anxious about issues of masculinity.*

Associations may at times be obvious and concrete (e.g., the city of Chicago above) or may be more abstract, but as a matter of technique it is best to hear the patient out before prematurely jumping to an interpretation.

Transference issues reflected in a dream. Dreams may be used to communicate feelings about the therapist and toward the therapeutic process. The patient may be unable to consciously recognize such feelings or too uncomfortable to state them directly; thus the dream is a disguised communication. In order for therapy to progress, the therapist must help the patient decode the message. The following clinical case illustrates how a patient early in therapy used the disguised language of a dream to express her feelings toward the therapist and the therapy itself.

> *A 25-year-old married woman and mother of two children began to see a therapist one week after her mother committed suicide by hanging. The patient's symptoms included anxiety, a fear that she might do something to harm herself, and the feeling that she was "walking on foam rubber or on a rocking boat." In the first few interviews she presented a torrid description of her sexual problems, including detailed confessions of premarital escapades. Interspersed with this material were expressions of fear that she would follow in her ill-fated mother's footsteps and of concern that her husband, who had money and time for his own pet hobbies but none for her, did not care about her. For the most part, however, current themes tended to be submerged. It was during her sixth hour, that the patient first reported a dream:*
>
> Patient: *I had this dream about the attic. . . . There was a man rummaging around up there. I didn't know what he was doing. There are a lot of things collected up there . . . from way back . . . things we don't use anymore. You know, things you save for no good reason, that you somehow just don't get around to throwing away—junk, old plumbing fixtures. I felt awfully uncomfortable with him being up there; I didn't know what to do. Then he left. It seemed as though he'd be back. [A minute of silence.] I suppose you'll be able to make something of that. Psychiatrists do that, don't they? Well?*
>
> Therapist: *Who was this man and what do you think he was doing up there?*
>
> Patient: *I just don't know. I never saw him before. I guess he knew what he was doing, but I sure didn't. He just came in and went right up there.*

Therapist: *Did you protest his invasion of your home?*

Patient: *Why, no. I seemed to know that he wanted to go up there. I even showed him the way to the attic stairs.*

Therapist: *Did you ask him to leave when you got uncomfortable?*

Patient: *No. I just felt I could not ask him to leave. I feel that I can't tell people what to do or not do. It was almost as if he had some business there or something. I just don't know. Isn't that ridiculous? After he left I crept up the attic stairs. I was afraid, but I just wanted to see. It looked as though he'd been rummaging around, particularly in the plumbing fixtures. There were even old toilets. They had been moved. And I even wondered whether he might have used them. And I expected him back!*

Therapist: *And you felt you'd let him go back up there?*

Patient: *Yes. How crazy can I get? It's a good thing it's just a dream.*

Therapist: *It seems as though you had him go up there in the first place—a kind of invitation almost?*

Patient: *I guess so. It seemed to be OK. I guess I didn't know what else to do.*

Therapist: *I'm the man in the attic.*

Patient: *[She looked thoughtful and blushed slightly.] That seems right. I don't know who else it could be. But what could you be doing in my attic?*

Therapist: *A better question might be: Why did you have me come up there? I think that the attic represents your accumulation of past memories about private, and especially sexual, experiences. I wonder if you feel that you are obliged to pour all these out to me as the "thing to do" when seeing a psychiatrist—that I expect this of you?*

Patient: *You do, don't you?*

There ensued a discussion concerning the importance of dealing with the problems that she herself felt were most pressing. The therapist who presented this account added the following note:

> *"I believe that the woman's use of the bathroom fixtures in a sense represents her feeling that I defiled her by letting her run on so much about her private experiences. These*

accounts were really quite inappropriate to the newness of our relationship and the nature of her needs at the time."

The dream as a condensation of the underlying conflict. Dreams, because of their fluidity in time and space, may serve to highlight central issues of conflict that may be condensed into a symbolic representation. The following case note illustrates this principle and also how it may be utilized in therapy.

> *A 25-year-old woman, wearing leg braces because of a disability dating back to her adolescent years, spent several hours complaining that it would be impossible for her to find a suitable mate. It was for this reason, she maintained, that she did not divorce her husband from whom she was legally separated. Each time she began to speak of something emotionally meaningful, tears welled up and she stopped. She felt there was no point in indulging in self-pity, and anyway she would surely come up against painful problems for which she would be unable to find solutions. She commented that men are only attracted to women who "play dumb and weak." Also, that women have to play up to men, and she could not because she found it impossible to be insincere and dishonest.*
>
> *The patient then recounted a dream she had the night before. In it she saw herself in a shower. She noticed that she had a penis that was so large that she would have to wear very long trousers to cover it. It was not hers but it was attached to her. The patient immediately thought of the trousers she wore to conceal her leg braces. Based on the dream, her association to it, and the context in which it occurred, the interpretation was made that because of her disability she felt unfeminine and, hence, unattractive to men she regarded as desirable. Thus, the interpretation, based partly on the dream, opened up an important area for scrutiny and discussion. It was evident that the patient tried to convince herself (and the therapist) that the attitude of men toward women was the stumbling block—that it was her unwillingness to play dumb and weak and not her physical disability that stood in the way. Following the interpretation of the dream, she began to examine her attitude toward her disability, especially the fact that it made her feel unfeminine.*

The following short dream is another example of how a dream can be used in psychotherapy.

> *During the hour previous to the dream, a young woman spoke of how she spent much time daydreaming during her unhappy childhood. She described her daydreams as being like Viennese waltzes or Victorian romances. The climax of the scene was a long tender first kiss. During this hour she recounted a dream in which water was leaking from the ceiling onto a couch. The couch in the dream was one in her apartment that she had purchased at a rummage sale. Water was actually leaking, and she moved her phonograph and some other pieces to protect them, but the couch was worth so little she did not bother to move it.*

She was silent for a few moments, and then she was unable to hold back a smile although she tried. Finally she said, "I suppose I should tell you the first thing that came to my mind. I haven't wanted to talk about it, but I have the feeling that I should." She then stated that she was thinking of how her man friend's penis was wet before he put on a condom. They had had intercourse on the couch shortly before she had the dream. She concluded that she must be the old couch.

These two pictures (perhaps among others) that she had of herself were pointed out: the Victorian, romantic and tender, and the other, sexual but like a cheap couch that is soiled. The two are companion pieces: one romantic and sexless; the other cheap and sexual. She responded by chuckling as she often did to an interpretation that was emotionally meaningful to her.

Long and/or detailed dreams. Long dreams present a special problem. The patient in spontaneous associations may dwell on certain parts and neglect others. It obviously is impractical to ask for associations to each part of the dream. The heart of the matter is selecting that portion which is most likely to yield "pay dirt." To an extent this is an intuitive matter. The therapist may be struck by a particular statement because of the flow of recent material, however, and conclude that it should be investigated. One rule of thumb is to look for the part of the dream that seems to refer to the treatment situation—to the relationship of patient and therapist—and inquire about it first. Another rule of thumb is to deal with context before content.

The following long dream will serve to demonstrate the manner in which a particular detail is initially selected.

> *A young man who had been in psychotherapy for approximately one year stated, "I had a dream Thursday*

night. I remember it now. I was going to visit someone. I was driving and I found that the brakes were bad again. Going down the hill, I kept making sharp turns to keep the car from gathering too much speed. I found a gas station with a woman mechanic. I thought that maybe I didn't have enough brake fluid. That once happened to me. A garage man said, 'No, it is not the fluid. There's a lot of work to be done.' The car was taken into a back room. There were lots of men in and around the car. I thought the men would be careless and abuse the car. There was an indoor ball game going on in the garage. A ball was hit and came down a track. I was in the way, and I didn't get out of the way soon enough. The man I interfered with was nice about it. It was 5:35 according to my watch. I worried about being late for supper. I thought my father would be angry. I asked the woman mechanic to drive me home. She was unwilling until I offered to pay her money. She consented. That's it."

The dream is rich in details and allusions and would appear even richer if the content of the preceding hours were cited, hours in which the patient spoke of embarrassing and frightening sexual experiences. This dream might be approached from any one of several points, but the portion that seemed most pertinent was: "A garage man said, 'No, it is not the fluid. There's a lot of work to be done.' "

When asked for his thoughts about this part of the dream, the patient mentioned the struggle he had gone through in recent hours. He hoped he was practically finished with the subject of sex, but somehow he felt that he was not. At this juncture it was pointed out to him that the garage man was really the therapist who was stating one of the patient's own views: namely, that there was a lot of work still to be done.

After dealing with the contextual matter—of reaching an understanding of the work still to be done—patient and therapist would then proceed to deal with the content: additional material of a sexual nature, the problem of controlling (faulty brakes) his penis (car). Parenthetically, it is significant that the patient had been enuretic and suffered from frequency and lack of control of urination in school as a child, had experienced guilt about masturbation as an adolescent, and made obscene phone calls to women as an adult.

The therapist's response to the dream. In the early days of psychoanalysis, Freud spent several hours working on a single dream. This procedure was soon abandoned and replaced by the approach of dealing with a dream only during the hour in which it was related unless the patient returned to it subsequently.

If special attention is focused on dreams (for example, if the therapist takes notes only when a dream is recounted), the patient is encouraged—or perhaps even conditioned—to communicate in the form of dreams. When this happens, the use of this means of communication rather than the content of the dreams themselves should be addressed. Many therapists contend that no special emphasis should be placed on dreams. It is difficult to avoid doing so, however, because dreams are such a rich source of information, and their unraveling, like decoding a message, is particularly fascinating.

One approach to dreams would be to regard them as the sleeper's way of thinking. Then it is assumed that the patient in dreaming would deal with unfinished business of the day. The issues to be dealt with may include conflicts and problems (Hollender 1962).

The patient's response to the dream. Although dreams usually serve to reveal feelings, they may also be used to disavow them. Not uncommonly, dreams are treated as though they are foreign bodies or belong to someone else. In other words, the productions of the unconscious are disowned. The patient must then be reminded, "This is your dream" or "You could have pictured things almost any way you chose, but this is the way you pictured them in *your* dream." A detached attitude toward dreams is especially common when patients write them down in detail and read them during the hour. The reading may sound like a report from a book, and for practical purposes this is what it is. To avoid falling into the trap of conducting an intellectual exercise about a third person, the therapist should point out the meaning of this behavior.

Dreams Used in Supportive Psychotherapy

Patients who are being treated with supportive psychotherapy on occasion report dreams. The dreams can often be used to disclose important information about the nature of the transference. Generally this type of information is not interpreted to the patient, although in certain situations, supportive interpretations may be deemed to be therapeutic (see Chapter 12). More often, the dream and the affect which accompanies it serve to reflect the patient's underlying mood. For example, a therapist should take note that a patient who reports a dream of wandering though a cemetery may be becoming more depressed.

Resistance

Resistance was defined by Freud (1900) as whatever interrupts the progress of the analytic work. According to Fenichel (1945), "Everything that prevents the patient from producing material derived from the unconscious is resistance." In the early years of psychoanalysis various methods were used to circumvent or overcome resistance, including pressure on the forehead accompanied by suggestion and insistence on forced concentration. Dream analysis and the rule of free association, which supplanted the earlier methods, were also mainly used to circumvent or overcome resistance. As attention shifted from id content to ego operations, resistance, while still regarded as an obstacle, also became a source of information.

The holdover of the picture of resistance as a roadblock has determined, in some measure, the persistence of the notion that it is necessary to go around or push through an obstacle. Such a viewpoint has determined and shaped the tactics of some therapists. Fenichel (1941), however, espoused a different approach.

> We obtain the desired effect upon the patient all the more lastingly and efficaciously if we succeed in using no other means of eliminating resistances than the confrontation of his reasonable ego with the fact of his resistance and the history of its origin.

The patient enmeshed in an intrapsychic struggle is likely to strive to convert the struggle into an interpersonal battle. It is easier to fight with someone else than with oneself. Not only should the therapist remain a noncombatant, but he or she should call attention to the patient's attempt to externalize one side of a struggle. The following clinical note illustrates this point.

> *A young man made two slips of the tongue. Each followed a brief silence and each was used as the basis for an interpretation. Following the next silence he expressed a reluctance to speak for fear he would make another slip that the therapist would "catch." It was suggested that he viewed*

> *the situation as one in which he might be caught off guard instead of one in which he would be helped to understand more about himself—that he regarded the therapist as an antagonist instead of a collaborator.*

The patient's struggle against facing unconscious impulses or wishes should remain an intrapsychic battle. It should not become "a kind of never-ending duel between the analyst and the patient's resistance" (Menninger 1961). By pointing out and describing resistances and their sources, the therapist becomes a collaborator with the nonresistant part of the patient in its struggle with the resistant part.

Regression

In classical psychoanalysis, regression is not only regarded as inevitable but also desirable (Macalpine 1950). The patient is expected to regress more and more deeply in the early phase and then to emerge later freed in large measure from conflicts or the mode of coping with them that had prompted the seeking of help. This thesis was stated clearly by Menninger (1961):

> Increasingly, in the course of treatment, he [the patient] will tend to "regress" to the lower levels; he will become more and more childlike in his attitude and in his emotional dependency upon the physician. He will become a child again, and be reborn, so to speak. Then he will grow up again, grow up better than he did before.

Regression, profound and sustained for therapeutic purposes, is essential only if one takes the viewpoint that reliving or reexperiencing childhood conflicts is a precondition for learning. With the introduction of ego psychology, the focus moved from the past to the here-and-now and from content to resistances. Accordingly, the patient's current behavior, in relationship to the therapist and others, has become the primary object of study. Patterns are discerned and examined, and later the origin of these patterns—or the old blueprints—are identified. To accomplish this, it is not necessary for the patient to regress and relive childhood conflicts. Those aspects of old conflicts important in adult life can be recognized in everyday feelings and in present behavior. For example, a man's problems with his father will be evident in his conduct with persons in authority, and, as would be expected, without profound regression they will be reexperienced in relationship to the therapist during psychotherapy.

The subject of regression has also been considered in another respect: in terms of the "desire to regress." It has been assumed by some therapists that a magnetic attraction pulls adults back toward a childlike state. According to this viewpoint, anyone given the opportunity will eagerly seek the gratification of being cared for and indulged by a parent-figure. No doubt some people will react in this manner, but the generalization is inaccurate and misleading. If regression were to occur at every opportunity, it would be necessary to frustrate patients to enlist their participation in psychotherapy. Also, such an orientation would fail to recognize the part played by the healthy part of the ego's desire for learning and mastery.

Summary

Dream analysis may be a useful, but by no means essential, projective technique that facilitates the acquisition of insight. Dreams, in certain respects, are similar to projective psychological tests, and therefore the effectiveness of their analysis depends both on the ability of the patient to generate this type of clinical material and the therapist's ability to correlate it with disparate aspects of the patient's life. As a general rule, the dream should be viewed first from the perspective of what it might say about the therapeutic relationship. With supportive techniques there is less emphasis on communicating new insights, but the dream may serve as a barometer of the patient's emotional state or as a means by which the therapist can better understand the patient's unconscious forces.

Resistance is viewed as demonstrating the patient's characteristic operations. The analysis and interpretation of resistance is a major part of treatment rather than an impediment to be overcome.

Regression is no longer regarded as a necessary condition for therapeutic change and, to the contrary, may interfere with the process of therapeutic work. Rather than promote conditions which facilitate regression, the therapist needs to engage the healthy part of the patient's ego to work actively toward the desired changes.

11

Time-Limited Insight-Oriented Psychotherapy

The length of time required for treatment has been of concern from the earliest days of psychoanalysis. Freud (1905a, 1905b) himself tended to be apologetic about the length of analyses even when they lasted only a few months. However, despite such concerns, the psychoanalytic establishment viewed with disfavor those analysts who experimented with differing techniques in their efforts to shorten treatment. Through the early decades of the twentieth century, the length of psychoanalytic treatment was gradually extended until analyses lasting several years were commonplace. Shorter forms of therapy were usually regarded as second rate, an approach to be used chiefly as an expedient measure—a psychological "Band-Aid."

The need for brief psychotherapies became more pressing after World War II. A greater appreciation of the importance of psychodynamic principles increased the demand on psychiatric services for psychotherapy. Concurrently there was the developing attitude that medical treatments should be available to all, not just the wealthy. More recently, there has been marked attention to the cost of delivering medical services with particular attention to psychotherapy. Questions of cost-effectiveness and cost accountability have been raised. Is long-term therapy more cost-effective than briefer therapies? Do the gains from psychotherapy justify their expense? Perhaps arbitrarily, insurance companies and governmental agencies have unilaterally made decisions to restrict their payment for psychotherapy. They have often limited their reimbursement to a finite number of sessions or have specified the limits of the number of sessions over a specific period of time (e.g., 20 sessions per year).

Historical Origins of Brief Psychotherapy

"Therapy was once short-term but it became longer and more complex; now the pendulum is swinging back, with the goal being shorter and more efficient treatment" (Budman and Stone 1983).

Among the pioneers working to reduce the length of dynamic psychotherapy were Alexander and French (1946). Recognizing the risk of overtreatment, they varied the frequency of sessions and set termination dates. Later, other innovations included shortening the length of the sessions and maintaining a high degree of focus on specific topics (Castelnuovo-Tedesco 1965).

Until the late 1960s, however, brief psychotherapy shared many characteristics of supportive psychotherapy. The emphasis was on symptom relief rather than enduring changes. The placebo effect and increased eclecticism, including the use of influence and suggestion, were emphasized as therapeutic techniques (Wolberg 1965). Such short-term psychotherapy with primary utilization of supportive techniques remains a common and well-accepted treatment modality. However, during the 1960s some clinicians began working, using selected patients, with time-limited insight-oriented psychotherapy. They had the more ambitious goals of altering long-standing maladaptive emotions, behavior, and cognitions. The continued progress of this work has been exciting.

Clinicians closely identified with the movement to include insight-oriented techniques in brief psychotherapy are Malan, Sifneos, Mann, Davanloo, and more recently Strupp and Binder. The underlying principles of patient selection and treatment for each of these proponents of time-limited therapy have many similarities as well as some distinctive characteristics.

The following discussion of time-limited insight-oriented psychotherapy represents a synthesis of those features for which there is a high degree of agreement. Differences, when important, will be noted. It must be emphasized that this chapter deals with time-limited psychotherapy in relation to insight-oriented or reconstructive psychotherapy. Supportive psychotherapy, also frequently used in a short-term manner, differs in many respects (see Chapter 12).

Definition and Description

Although brief forms of psychotherapy were initially developed in an effort to reduce the length of time required for treatment, the resultant therapeutic approach in some instances was more than merely an abridgement: It was a distinctive approach especially well suited to the treatment of patients with particular types of psychopathology.

Short-term dynamic psychotherapy has been defined and described as

> . . . a treatment modality in which a single conflict underlying a patient's main complaint or symptom is focused upon actively and tenaciously during a series of weekly vis-à-vis sessions, usually numbering 12 to 20, with an upper limit of 30. Psychodynamic principles are used to understand and trace the focal conflict back to its origin. Transference attitudes and distortions related to the focal conflict are confronted actively as they arise. (Weissberg 1984)

Selection of Patients for Time-Limited Psychotherapy

A major consideration in the use of an insight-oriented technique in conjunction with a time limitation is the accurate identification of patients who will benefit from this approach. Features of brief psychotherapy associated with a favorable outcome have probably received more attention from investigators than have those associated with other approaches. This is most likely due to the fact that it is easier to measure outcome in shorter than in longer forms of therapy.

Criteria for selection for time-limited psychotherapy originally were quite stringent. As greater experience has been acquired with this technique, the criteria have been relaxed. Selection criteria now minimize diagnosis and presenting symptoms and focus more on characteristics specifically related to the problems anticipated. Characteristics suggesting a favorable outcome are at times found in patients who, on the surface, have serious psychopathology as indicated by their diagnoses. Factors that essentially all investigators and clinicians would emphasize as having importance in the selection of patients for time-limited insight-oriented psychotherapy include the following:

1. The capacity to establish a relationship with the therapist. The patient must be able to engage and interact quickly with the therapist. This ability can be judged by the quality of the relationship during the evaluation period and inferred from the patient's history of interpersonal relationships in both the present and the past.

2. An identifiable focal conflict. Short-term therapy is ineffective if the patient's problems are diffuse and there is no central organizing focus of attention. By the end of the evaluation period, both the therapist and patient should be able to agree on a psychodynamic formulation; in a few paragraphs it should be possible to tell the story of the patient's major problem or conflict and explain it with psychodynamic concepts.

3. Adequate ego strength. The patient must possess sufficient ego strength to be able to tolerate the inevitable anxiety or depression mobilized by the intensity of the treatment process. Patients who characteristically react to frustration with regression or serious acting out (e.g., suicidal gestures) are not likely to be candidates for this approach. Ego strength can be estimated by the patient's responses to prior life stressors.

4. Motivation. The importance of motivation cannot be overestimated. Patients must want to get better and be willing to work on problems not only during treatment hours but also between them.

5. Psychological mindedness. The patient must have some capacity to link affects, behavior, and prior experiences. Included in this quality of "psychological mindedness" is the ability to see oneself as having responsibility for one's own feelings and behavior rather than projecting this responsibility on another person (e.g., a spouse). The potential for working with psychological concepts can be tested by responses to trial interpretations made during the evaluation period. Did the patient react by providing new and confirmatory information? Was there an insightful reflection on the ideas presented? If the evaluation period extended over more than one session, did differences in the two sessions indicate that the patient had reflected and worked on material discussed during the first hour?

According to Marmor (1979), two patient selection factors are especially relevant to and essential for a short-term psychotherapeutic approach. The first is the existence of a *focal conflict.* During the first interview, or the first two at the most, the therapist should be able to identify a central conflictual problem around which most of the patient's difficulties revolve. The other selection factor of prime importance for short-term therapy is the existence of a clear-cut and strong motivation to change. The critical issue is not diagnosis but the possession of certain personality attributes plus the existence of a focal conflict and a high level of motivation.

Techniques

The basic principles of insight-oriented psychotherapy are as appropriate for time-limited therapy as they are for more prolonged therapies. The therapist does not impose his or her value system on the patient, and the concepts of self-determination and personal responsibility are not altered. The therapist continues to search for and decode unconscious messages by whatever means are available, including dreams. There is, however, far less emphasis on "free association" because of the need to maintain both the working alliance and the focus on the central conflict. The following technical operations are distinguishing characteristics of time-limited insight-oriented psychotherapy.

1. Determining the length of therapy. With brief psychotherapy, a primary tenet is that the treatment will be "time-limited"; therapy will have a finite length. How is the length determined? Different authors have advocated various ways. Mann (1973) proposed an arbitrary 12 sessions for all patients. Most other authors permit somewhat greater flexibility. At the Tavistock Clinic, Malan (1980) set a general limit of 30 sessions for most therapies but indicated that, for those patients with a favorable outcome, the mean was usually 20 sessions. Moreover, he advocated setting a termination date rather than assigning a predetermined number of sessions.

Sifneos (1972) makes it clear to patients during the evaluation that psychotherapy is expected to last only a few months but no specific number of sessions or termination date is stated. Interviews of 45 minutes duration are held weekly, and most treatments last 12 to 16 sessions with no more than 20. Davanloo (1979) recommended a treatment length from five to 40 sessions depending on the nature of the patient's conflict area. In general his therapies require 15 to 25 sessions. He does not recommend setting a specific termination date but rather indicating to the patient that treatment will be short. Strupp and Binder (1986) strongly advocated that the time limit be set after a therapeutic focus has begun to be outlined by the participants "because the introduction of a focus is more likely to provide the patient with a belief that there are circumscribed goals that can be achieved in the available time."

We favor an approach in which the length of treatment is set at the end of the evaluation. To set it before knowing about the nature of the patient's problems would indicate that the patient's problems must be trimmed to the treatment rather than vice versa. Similarly, failure to set a limit until midway into therapy in some ways undercuts the entire principle of time-limited psychotherapy. It introduces the possibility that the termination date may be determined less by the needs of the patient or the therapeutic goals and more by countertransference issues that have arisen. After evaluating the nature of the patient's problem, the focal conflict should be identified. The length of time needed to resolve the conflict should be estimated and a termination date set.

2. Activity by the therapist. In time-limited psychotherapy, the therapist does not have the luxury of passivity, waiting for dynamic materials to demonstrate their validity repeatedly before reacting with confrontations and interpretations. Rather, the confrontations and interpretations must come early in the course of therapy and, consequently, they are often based on less than solid evidence. Such interventions require intuition and experience. Because of these factors, therapists with much experience in long-term psychotherapy will size up situations more rapidly and will be able to make accurate interpretations at an earlier point in therapy.

Because of the time limit, the therapist must constantly be vigilant, looking for dynamic material relevant either to the central conflict or the transference that may have an impact on therapy. This type of activity is perhaps best typified by Davanloo (1979), who was self-described as the "relentless healer." He actively and repetitively confronted the patient in order to break through characterological defenses.

3. Maintenance of the therapeutic alliance. The therapist must remember that therapy progresses through the mutual work of therapist and patient. Regressive tendencies on the part of the patient should be discouraged. Patients may need to be reminded that the therapist cannot solve their problems for them and that magical expectations are unrealistic.

4. Therapeutic focus on the central conflict. Successful short-term insight-oriented psychotherapy is highly dependent on resolution of and increased capability to deal with the central conflict. Patients may repetitively attempt digressions, many of which will be intellectually interesting. The danger is that the therapist will be seduced into following the patient's lead. However, such temptations should be withstood, and the patient must be actively reminded of the details of the original therapeutic contract. Such interpretations of resistance inevitably elicit anxiety and/or hostile feelings toward the therapist. However, it is the capacity to tolerate such difficulties in therapy that led to the selection of this treatment technique for particular patients.

5. Active interpretation of the transference. In discussing transference interpretations in focal psychotherapy (a time-limited therapy in which the emphasis is placed on the circumscribed nature of the psychopathology), Frances and Perry (1983) stated that transference interpretations are appropriate in the following circumstances: 1) when feelings have become the point of urgency or a major resistance; 2) when transference distortions have disrupted the therapeutic alliance and interpretations are necessary to strengthen the alliance; 3) when conflicts revealed in the transference directly reflect conflicts responsible for the presenting problem or maladaptive character traits; 4) when the patient has the psychological-mindedness to observe, understand, tolerate, and apply transference interpretations; and 5) when the length of remaining treatment will allow sufficient exploration of whatever transference interpretations are made.

Frances and Perry (1983) also described the situations in which transference interpretations may be unnecessary or not advised: 1) the patient does not develop strong or apparent transference distortions; 2) the point of emotional urgency and the related intrapsychic conflicts are fixed on current events and relationships outside the treatment situation; 3) a fragile therapeutic alliance will be jeopardized further by a distressing and unacceptable transference interpretation; 4) the patient does not have the psychological mindedness to observe, understand, tolerate, and use transference interpretations; 5) transference distortions are not related clearly enough to the presenting problem or to significant maladaptive character traits; and 6) remaining treatment time is too limited for even a partial analysis of transference material.

An example of the type of transference distortion that would block progress in treatment is that of a patient who had realized that her feelings of being unworthy were based on relationships with significant others in her past. The authors (Frances and Perry 1983) stated, "Through the analysis of her misperceptions of the therapist, she could simultaneously correct the way she perceived and related to her boyfriends and [her] family. In the therapist's judgment, interpretations of the transference were not only indicated but unavoidable."

6. *Keeping the termination date.* The patient may exert strong pressure to change the termination date and to prolong treatment to avoid the pain of separation and loss. However, the very act of setting the termination date has provoked these feelings, and the continuous anticipation of the end of therapy tends to propel therapeutic progress. Continuous renegotiation of the termination date would create a situation similar to that of the parent who has difficulty setting limits for children and repeatedly renegotiates the rules of conduct. Therefore, the termination date, once set, should not be changed unless there are extremely compelling reasons to do so. If there is to be a change, the entire therapeutic contract should be renegotiated with the establishment of new goals and new ground rules. At such times, it may be advisable to refer the patient to another therapist with whom a different type of therapeutic alliance and a new therapeutic contract can be established.

In discussing the technique for short-term dynamic psychotherapy, Marmor (1979) listed general and specific factors. The general factors common to all dynamic therapies included 1) catharsis in a setting of hope and the expectation of help, 2) a constructive patient-therapist relationship, 3) cognitive learning based on interpretations, 4) operant conditioning based on indications of the therapist's approval or disapproval, 5) identification with the therapist, 6) elements of suggestion and persuasion, and 7) some aspects of practice and rehearsal of new adaptive techniques and their generalization.

The four specific factors cited by Marmor (1979) were that 1) the patient is always seen sitting up and facing the therapist; 2) a time limit is always involved, which from the beginning places a central emphasis on the issues of separation and individuation; 3) a persistent focus is maintained throughout on the core conflict and defensive digressions from that central focus are not permitted; and 4) the activity of the therapist, consisting of persistent confrontations and interpretations, serves to discourage regression.

A Clinical Example

The following case report will illustrate several of the points made in the preceding sections of this chapter.

> *A 22-year-old man stated that he was seeking advice. He wished to remain in his family's business, but to do so he had to live in a small and remote village, and this he found intolerable. In discussing his motives for entering the family business, he mentioned the pledge he had made to himself six years before when he first learned that his father and mother had been killed in a plane crash. He described a strong sense of obligation to carry on for his father and also a desire thereby to perpetuate his relationship with him. The same feeling of obligation led him to assume the role of the oldest brother, although actually he was the middle of three sons. In doing so, it seemed he had pushed aside many of his own needs and had grown up ahead of his time.*
>
> *It quickly became evident that intense feelings of loss had been bottled up, and it took only a few questions to bring them out. The focus then shifted from the current conflict to unresolved feelings of loss. (The latter clearly seemed to be related to the former.)*
>
> *The patient stated that he had cried for his parents only once and that was at the graveside when everyone else except the minister had left. He next spoke of the period of five days that passed before the wreckage of the plane and the bodies of his parents were finally found. During that time, and even to an extent ever since, he thought of them as still being alive and he continued to look for them in crowds.*
>
> *As the patient spoke of his devastating sense of loss and the longing to see his father and mother, he began to cry quietly, and it was several minutes before he could resume his account. He then stated that perhaps the therapist was correct in suggesting that he had not mourned his loss.*
>
> *It was recommended that the patient be seen for six sessions at weekly intervals and that the focus be on the delayed mourning reaction. The recommendation was readily accepted.*
>
> *At the second appointment, the patient stated that he was aware that his work situation had merely served to bring feelings about his parents to the surface. When they were killed, they were returning from a visit with their oldest son,*

who was hospitalized for a mental illness, but the patient did not think he blamed his brother. During the weekend before his second appointment, a dog that his parents had purchased was put to sleep. The patient was aware that he needed to see and touch the pet for a sense of finality, a feeling he had not had with his parents because of the closed caskets at the funeral.

At his third appointment, the patient returned to feelings about his older brother, stating that he thought his brother should have felt guilty about their parents' deaths. When it was suggested that he blamed his brother, he agreed but stated that obviously he should not. When the aunt with whom he went to live after his parents' deaths tried to be a mother to him, he resented it. He felt, "How dare she try to take my mother's place?" It was also pointed out that he felt that she was calling on him to be disloyal. He had not realized this, but he thought it was true. At the time of the tragedy, the patient had a "peculiar feeling"—a feeling of being relieved because what he had feared would happen, he need dread no longer. It was suggested that this feeling stemmed from the fact that he had not caused the accident, that he was not responsible for the deaths of his parents as he feared he might be. He responded that perhaps he had been concerned about his angry feelings; he had engaged in an intense argument with his mother shortly before she left to visit his brother.

By the sixth and final appointment, the patient was more at peace about his work situation, because he no longer felt that he was required to remain in the family business. The decision was his to make. He also commented that now when he thought about his parents, he no longer experienced a "stabbing feeling in his gut." During the previous few weeks he dated a young woman, and he mentioned, "She is the first one who doesn't resemble my mother."

In this instance the patient's presenting complaint was a conflict, focal in nature, that he was unable to resolve. The relationship of the conflict to a delayed grief reaction was quickly discerned. His ego strength seemed more than adequate and motivation was strong. The approach recommended was time-limited—six weekly appointments. The initial focus was on the delayed grief reaction and its bearing on the current conflict.

Summary

With selected patients, time-limited insight-oriented psychotherapy can be an exciting endeavor, gratifying both for the patient and the therapist. In addition to the relief of anxiety and depression, dramatic changes can occur in a patient's ways of handling certain conflictual issues. To paraphrase Sifneos (1984), it is difficult not to like such patients when one witnesses how hard they work, and how motivated they are to face and resolve their difficulties despite the anxiety that therapy tends to arouse in them.

12

Supportive Psychotherapy

Of all of our therapeutic modalities, supportive psychotherapy is the most widely used and the least uniformly taught. All too often it is assumed that good intentions and everyday intuition are all that is required. Consequently, it is not unusual to tell beginning clinical trainees to provide supportive psychotherapy and then cut them loose with little or no supervision. Although the help that they may provide patients should not be denigrated, there is a difference between being supportive and applying the principles of supportive psychotherapy in a skillful and systematic manner with specific objectives and goals in mind.

Questions raised in discussing supportive psychotherapy include the following: "For whom is this form of treatment indicated?" "What is being supported?" and "What are the specific techniques employed to provide the desired support?" These questions will be addressed in this chapter.

Supportive psychotherapy is similar to insight-oriented psychotherapy in that both are built on the therapist's understanding of the patient's psychodynamics. They differ, however, in how that understanding is used. In supportive psychotherapy, the therapist's knowledge of the patient's psychodynamic structure may shape the therapeutic approach but seldom serves as the basis for interpretations.

The goal is to strengthen defenses, restore the previous psychological homeostasis, reduce anxiety, and increase the tolerance for unalterable situations (Conte and Plutchik 1986). For acute disorders the objective is likely to be the restoration of an equilibrium, and for chronic disorders bolstering the patient whenever and wherever the need arises. In both situations, the development of a positive transference is fostered, observed, and used; an effort is made to eliminate a negative transference if it appears.

Indications for Supportive Psychotherapy

Supportive psychotherapy is the treatment of choice when external pressures threaten to be overwhelming or when internal resources are severely limited by ego weakness or defect. Advanced age and impaired physical condition frequently favor the use of supportive measures.

The decision to employ supportive techniques as the primary therapeutic strategy must be based, as is the case with all types of psychotherapy, on the findings of the evaluation and an understanding of the psychodynamics involved.

The evaluation and formulation should take into account 1) the patient's ego strength and weakness, 2) recent losses or other stressors that may have resulted in a reduction of self-esteem, 3) the nature of defense mechanisms and the degree that they may be helpful or harmful in coping with stress, 4) the extent that intoxicating chemicals affect the current level of functioning, and 5) the highest level of functioning previously achieved and the circumstances.

From the evaluation, certain principles evolve that can be employed in treatment planning. Among these are the axiom that the most basic functions must be supported best, for example reality testing in the psychotic patient or the preservation of life in a despondent, severely depressed patient. It is unlikely that psychotherapy of any type can be effective in the face of ongoing substance abuse and this must be addressed directly. It is also unrealistic to expect patients to reach a higher level of functioning than they had achieved in the past. Therefore, one treatment strategy is to help them reinstitute the life circumstances, including the coping mechanisms, associated with their highest level of previous functioning.

Techniques

Specific techniques utilized in supportive psychotherapy have been described by various authors. We have selected those that are most readily definable, while keeping in mind that there are also nonspecific aspects of treatment (Strupp and Hadley 1979; Karasu 1986) and that many of the techniques overlap to some degree.

As a general rule, the therapist in this kind of therapy needs to be relatively active but without crowding the patient. Dependency should be accepted to an appreciable extent but kept within workable limits by controlling the frequency and length of sessions and telephone calls. For some patients, setting a definite length of time for therapy in advance may be helpful. The effect of psychotherapy may also be augmented by the use of medication, or treatment may consist primarily of manipulation, direct or indirect, of the patient's environment.

Among the other technical procedures commonly employed, singly or in combinations, are catharsis, suggestion, persuasion, advice-giving, reassurance, and direction. The actual expression of support may take many forms, most of them verbal but a significant number nonverbal. The latter range from facial expressions showing empathy and concern to offering a tissue to a crying patient.

The following approaches are among those that serve to bolster patients in supportive psychotherapy.

Enhancement of Self-Esteem

Many patients who are candidates for supportive psychotherapy suffer from acute blows to their self-esteem (recent marital separation would be an example) or chronic blows (lack of occupational success would be an example). Feelings of self-worth and a sense of dignity may be enhanced by the therapist's genuine respect, concern, and regard for the patient and an empathic understanding of the patient's plight and suffering. This approach stands in sharp contrast to the use of Pollyannish statements like "Everything will turn out for the best" or superficial praise like "My, how well you look today."

The following case note is one in which self-esteem played a central role.

> *The members of Mr. N's family were immobilized. They had been advised to commit him to the local state hospital for his own safety, but they stood in awe of him and were afraid of possible repercussions. Mr. N had been a powerful figure in the community for forty years, the head of one of the largest corporations and a prominent and much respected social leader. But he had begun to drink to excess, and when inebriated he would engage in target practice in his basement. Not only was the family concerned about ricocheting bullets, but they were afraid of what he might do next. Finally, they asked him to see a psychiatrist, and they were amazed and relieved that he was willing.*

Mr. N looked the part of the successful industrialist. His presence was commanding, and his manner of speaking was theatrical. After talking about the kind of life he had lived—as a pilot in World War I, as a person who sought out danger in athletics and hunting, and as a man who welcomed and met challenges—he talked about the heart attack he had experienced three months before. He explained that the heart attack left him feeling like his "sword was broken." (One hardly need be a Freudian to recognize the symbolism.) Previously he had been in excellent health. Now he had difficulty falling asleep and drank, sometimes almost to the point of stupor, to overcome the effects of depression and anxiety that interfered with sleep.

The therapist did not find it difficult to genuinely admire Mr. N and to convey that feeling to him. As the patient reestablished his sense of manliness, he cut back on his drinking and gave up target practice. After six months of weekly appointments, the sessions were "spaced and spanned" and then discontinued. According to a report received from a member of his family, he functioned well until his death about five years later.

The main component of Mr. N's successful therapy consisted of his ability to reconceptualize himself as a strong man. This was achieved in considerable measure through the therapist's admiration of his past accomplishments and by the patient's vicariously reliving earlier successes.

The Therapist as an Authority

The special position occupied in our society by physicians and other professional therapists may be used to produce a desired effect. As the authority on psychological matters, the therapist's statements carry extra weight and therefore may be supportive. The following case note is illustrative.

The old thesis that doing the least is best sometimes applies to psychotherapy. Such seemed to be true in the case of Mrs. E, a 46-year-old woman who was turning to a psychiatrist for the first time. Fifteen years before, she had developed the notion that people were talking about her, accusing her of trying to involve men at the church she attended in sexual activity. This notion faded considerably after she talked about it a few times with her husband and the pastor. During the next few years, when it threatened to reemerge, she was able to convince herself that people were not really saying what she thought they were saying.

Mrs. E called—from a pay phone—for an appointment in the psychiatric clinic when the accusations she overheard became so loud and insistent that she could no longer push them aside. They had become so upsetting that she considered suicide but had not yet formulated a specific plan. She hoped that a physician with special knowledge and training would be able to be of more help now than her husband and pastor could be. A well-dressed, fairly attractive, and pleasant woman, Mrs. E clearly considered it important to be agreeable and likable. Her use of reaction formations to cope with hostility was transparent. The psychologist who tested her discerned that she had glaring problems in dealing with hostility and sexuality. Mrs. E described her own marriage as good. Two daughters were married, and a third daughter was in college.

It seemed likely that Mrs. E would be able to use the authority of the physician-psychiatrist to fortify her in her struggle to keep unacceptable feelings submerged or, at least, in check for a time. She was seen for three appointments, and the anticipated result was achieved.

The Therapist's Empathy

For a patient, to be understood is likely to be experienced as being supported. Accordingly, if the therapist is able to resonate with the patient, a meaningful degree of comfort will be afforded. The therapist's understanding is especially important when family and friends fail to comprehend the patient's plight and struggle.

To a depressed patient, the therapist, based on what he or she hears or infers, may comment that the patient apparently thinks this episode is the worst ever. If this statement is confirmed, the therapist might add, "No doubt you find it very difficult to think back to a time when you felt well, and you find it even more difficult to think that you will ever feel like your old self again—but you will."

The therapist also shows understanding in commenting on the patient's work performance: "I know you are not performing up to par; a depressed person rarely does. It may even have gone so far that routine tasks, tasks you formerly did with hardly a thought, now seem so large that they almost look insurmountable."

Here again, the therapist gives reassurance, even though he or she is aware that the patient's pessimistic outlook makes it difficult to share the therapist's confidence that the present symptoms are transitory. Some pressure may be relieved if the patient can accept the therapist's assurance that the problem with concentration and the diminution or loss of libido will recede as the depression recedes. Finally, the patient needs to be reminded now and again that anyone who is depressed sees almost everything through dark colored glasses.

The person who feels understood does not stand alone. Hence, the therapist's demonstration of empathy is a fundamental building block in supportive psychotherapy.

Promotion of Therapeutic Optimism

Many patients who are demoralized and pessimistic express feelings of helplessness and hopelessness. Yet, if they voluntarily seek treatment, it can be assumed that they harbor at least some hope of being helped. The initiation of the relationship with a therapist, as a general rule, carries with it positive feelings, much as the sick child is comforted by the presence of the parent. The task of the therapist is to do nothing that will undermine this inherently beneficial quality of the doctor-patient relationship. The professional role should be maintained by dress and manner, projecting a quiet confidence in one's skills and expressing therapeutic concern. These nonverbal messages, interpreted by the patient as reassurance of being in competent hands, carry with them the anticipation of being helped.

Promotion of Reality Testing

Patients may sometimes misinterpret environmental events, other persons' motivations, and their own sensations. Although it is futile to attempt to convince a person that he or she is delusional, skillful questioning and comments may help the patient to focus on reality issues in the here-and-now. This can be done partially by behavioral modification techniques such as failing to respond to irrelevant or psychotic material and instead redirecting to or reinforcing discussions of real issues. At times a therapist may respond to what appears to be a patient's faulty perception with a question such as "Have you considered alternative explanations such as . . . ?"

Problem Solving

Patients are frequently beset with multiple external stressors that appear to call for some form of decision making or action. The therapist may encourage the patient to weigh carefully the possible consequences of various courses of action and suggest that there are often multiple alternatives. It may also be appropriate to suggest that some decisions should be deferred until the patient is better able to deal with problems (e.g., financial decisions when hypomanic, depressed, or cognitively impaired). Such an approach may not only result in better decisions but may also be a learning experience for the impulse-ridden or disorganized person. One must be careful, however, not to reinforce procrastination that perpetuates or reinforces passive-aggressive behavior.

Providing Advice

There is a definite place for advice, but care must be taken that it is offered in the context of the patient's value system (unless antisocial) and not as an imposition of the therapist's values. A relatively noncontroversial type of advice would be to strongly urge someone with legal problems (e.g., a potential divorce) to seek the services of an attorney. Another noncontroversial type of advice would be to urge or insist that someone with physical symptoms that might indicate a serious disease seek the services of a medical specialist. Areas that might be more controversial would be recommending that a lonely and socially isolated person join a church or synagogue. Still more controversial would be advice to initiate divorce proceedings.

There are two major concerns with giving advice: 1) the advice may be poor because no one is omniscient or because the patient may have misrepresented the facts, and 2) giving advice often has a regressive effect; responsibility is shifted from the patient to the therapist.

We shall explore one of the more common forms of advice—urging a person to take a vacation. (Similar advice is to tell a person to remain away from work or school for a period of time.) The advice to take a vacation may be given too freely because it is regarded as innocuous, the "aspirin" of nonmedicinal prescriptions. Although vacationing is undoubtedly beneficial for some patients, it may have undesirable "side-effects" for others.

Symptoms that seem to be due to external pressure are sometimes really due to internal tension. Such was the case for a man treated by Levine (1947), whose insomnia and fatigue were attributed to overwork. When the patient acted on his physician's advice to take a vacation in Florida, his symptoms became more intense. Only then was it learned that his distress had not been caused by overwork but by a conflict about his impulses to be unfaithful to his wife. The tempting sight of attractive women in scanty swimwear on the beach increased his conflict and his tension.

Some patients told to get away from it all, to go where they can have a good time and rest up, are the ones who might commit suicide. "They are the ones whose inner fears cause them to go to a physician looking for support, and instead they are sent off to a strange environment where there is no one to lend them support" (Barhash 1951).

Persons who are very dependent on work to maintain their emotional balance are likely to set up a seven-day-a-week schedule and even have a second job. If, in spite of this schedule, they do not succeed in staving off tension-produced symptoms, it would seem incorrect to assume that overwork is the culprit and that a vacation should be prescribed. Such a prescription is likely to work in reverse, with the result being intensified distress.

A rough measure of how a person will react to a vacation can be obtained by exploring the response to time off work on weekends and holidays. If the response is favorable, a prescription for a vacation may prove effective. If it is unfavorable, such a prescription is not likely to be effective and may even be contraindicated. Persons who avoid time off or do poorly when unoccupied have been described as having a "Sunday neurosis," an anxiety reaction generated by unacceptable impulses that threaten to erupt when attention is not engaged by outside activity.

Catharsis or Ventilation

Dysphoric feelings such as anger, frustration, or depression may be bottled up. With ventilation there is a feeling of relief and often of increased comfort. Such improvement, however, is often transient because the underlying conflict remains unresolved. For example, a wife may feel better while angrily complaining about her husband, but her expressions of anger in therapy will not alter the underlying unsatisfactory marital relationship. Catharsis or ventilation may produce more long-lasting therapeutic gains in situations such as grief, where the expression of emotions may facilitate the mourning process. In other situations, ventilation may be the preferable alternative to an open expression of emotion (e.g., anger) in a situation that cannot be altered. And, finally, an open expression of feelings may be the first step in acknowledgment of previously repressed, constricted, or inhibited affects. One contraindication to the free expression of emotions is encountered in the patient with a histrionic or borderline personality who characteristically gives full vent to emotional expression.

Reduction of Feelings of Loneliness and Isolation

Although "purchased" in one sense, supportive psychotherapy does provide a genuine human relationship and the opportunity to share feelings and ideas with another person. Psychotherapy, therefore, assists in providing some auxiliary social support for persons who feel a sense of disconnectedness.

In the following case note, loneliness and isolation were significant factors.

> *Mrs. K, a 73-year-old married woman, was seen for evaluation of a long-standing depression. Tricyclic antidepressant medication, prescribed by her internist, had been somewhat effective in reducing her physiologic symptoms but her mood remained depressed. She felt lonely, isolated, and useless. Her retired physician husband left daily to play golf with cronies and her only daughter, who occasionally asked her to babysit, was busy with her career and spent little time with her mother.*
>
> *Mrs. K was seen for 30 minutes every other week in supportive psychotherapy. The therapist listened with genuine interest to stories of her childhood in pre-World War II Czechoslovakia. She spoke with pride of her father, a railroad official, and her enjoyment of the train trips they took together.*
>
> *Mrs. K had difficulty in dealing directly with her feelings. A pattern emerged in which she expressed herself indirectly by occasionally bringing small gifts to the therapist. Each was carefully chosen and had meaning. For example, a recording of Horowitz (then 76 years old) playing piano encore selections set the theme of one 30-minute session. Although the personal meaning of the gift was never explicitly stated, namely, that an elderly person might continue to have talents and be of value in society, it seemed to be understood.*
>
> *Therapy was successful in that Mrs. K's mood brightened. She made her therapy sessions the high point of her week, and she planned her visits so that her hair was*

> *dressed and other activities were arranged along with her trip to the therapist. A positive transference was obvious but not interpreted. When the first therapist moved away, a direct referral was made to another therapist, and Mrs. K was able to transfer her positive feelings to the second therapist who continued to use the same general approach with equal success.*

The components of successful supportive psychotherapy with this woman included 1) an empathic acceptance of her as an aging person; 2) recognizing and helping her obtain pleasure from recollections of more pleasant and successful periods of her life; 3) providing a focus for her energies and a sense of pride in selecting gifts for the therapist (issues around gifts to a therapist can be very complex and accepting gifts from some patients may be contraindicated; see Chapter 14); and 4) decreasing her isolation and loneliness, thus providing social interaction and, in addition, a reason for associated activities.

Clarification

Patients who seek help because of feelings of anxiety, depression, anger, or a sense of losing control may have difficulty separating the real issues from a variety of "straw men." The therapist may assist in disentangling these constructs and thereby make it possible to reach better decisions. For example, a woman might rail at conditions at her workplace when the real issue is her resentment at having to work when she would prefer to be at home with her children.

Praise

The idea that a therapist can shape behavior through the use of rewards or extinguish it through benign neglect may be anathema to many persons. There is, however, little doubt that either consciously or unconsciously therapists provide their patients with feedback indicating either approval or disapproval of certain behavior or affects. Patients may be motivated to make changes, take chances, and allow more expression of affect if they think that they are pleasing their therapists. Although praise may significantly interfere with the process of insight-oriented psychotherapy, it may, when judiciously used, be an important component of supportive psychotherapy.

Repression of Unacceptable Emotions or Ideas

Often it is mistakenly assumed that it is beneficial to "let it all hang out" or that the uncensored expression of ideas has therapeutic benefit. Unfortunately, this often is not the case, and the therapist is well advised to help the patient "keep the lid on." Patients with limited ego strength, who experience frequent eruptions of primary process thinking accompanied by disorganization, benefit when the therapist maintains a structured, reality-based interaction. The therapist may need to intervene often to redirect discussions to practical and goal-oriented issues. For these patients, encouraging free association and the expression of fantasies is contraindicated.

Similarly many patients, and in particular those with borderline disorders or histrionic personality traits, have difficulty in appropriately modulating their affects. Their histrionic behavior and emotional storms need to be tempered. This can be done subtly by a failure to respond to the affect (extinction) or by more direct statements that the patient's affect is counterproductive: "It isn't helpful to continue to be so angry about something that can't be changed."

Reduction of Stress

The removal of pressure may have a dramatic effect when external stress is largely responsible for a state of emotional decompensation. The removal may be achieved by discussing the situation, as in the case described below, or it may be achieved by direction with or without an explanation. When an overburdened patient cannot unburden himself or herself because doing so would produce guilt, it is often necessary to deal with the guilt before the problem can be resolved.

The following case (Miller 1957) is one in which a supportive approach consisted of removing the stressor responsible for a state of decompensation. In this instance, as often occurs, the pressure was manifested in the form of bodily complaints—what was not expressed in words was expressed as symptoms.

> *Mr. M, an unsmiling, humorless, 46-year-old mechanic, stated in an indifferent fashion that he had cancer. He complained of swollen glands in his axilla and of pain in the jaw. He felt sure the bones in his face were "deteriorating." To find out the truth, he had taken a leave of absence from his job. Discussion with the patient revealed that he had*

developed his symptoms in the face of long-continuing and growing pressure from his fiancée to end their engagement with marriage. In the face of this pressure to take responsibility for that which he felt totally inadequate, he had become increasingly tense, developed headaches, and discovered normal-sized lymph glands, which he mistakenly believed were cancerous. He avoided his fiancée and spent increasingly more time worrying about the possibility of cancer. Subsequent discussion with him about his feelings concerning the impending marriage led to its indefinite postponement. The symptoms subsided, and he returned to work.

Incidental Assistance

In some instances in which patients do not respond favorably to pharmacotherapy or psychotherapy or a combination of the two, it may still be possible to provide support.

A middle-aged woman, who suffered from recurrent bouts of depression that were refractory to treatment, would consistently attribute her discomfort to something her husband did or did not do. Because of her anger she could not turn to him for help. When her pattern of blaming him was scrutinized and discussed, it became possible for her to see him as an ally rather than as an enemy. This made the situation somewhat more tolerable for both of them.

When this same patient was able, with some prompting from the therapist, to tell her teenaged daughter and son that she had an illness and that their behavior was not the cause of her unhappiness, some of the tension in the home situation was relieved.

Supportive Interpretations

Most therapists sharply separate insight-oriented and supportive psychotherapy. Pine (1986) does not. He maintains that the two approaches are by no means inconsistent with one another, and that most supportive treatments include some exploratory and interpretive work. The distinction drawn between the interpretation given in insight-oriented and supportive psychotherapy is that the former is given in the context of abstinence and the latter in the context of support.

The following example was cited by Pine (1986):

> In an *explanatory* and *sympathetic* tone the therapist may say something like: "You know Mr. Ames, as I listen to you I realize that (such and such—the interpretation) is true of you. I understand that it frightens you and that you don't like to think of yourself as having such thoughts. But most people have them, and we can work together later on to help you so you can get a handle on them." Many supportive statements are included in this intervention. The therapist has made explicit his or her nonjudgmental and helpful stance.

The following is another example cited by Pine: "I'm not sure about this idea; I'd like you to tell me what you think. It occurred to me that (and the interpretation is given). Does that sound possible to you?" The patient is given the opportunity in advance to accept or reject the interpretation.

In those instances, probably relatively few in number, in which interpretations are offered in therapy that is primarily supportive, support should be provided in words and reassurance should be provided in tone. Moreover, Pine stated,

> When the therapist decides that the patient simply cannot deal with interpretation at the "hot" moment, it may be useful to delay . . . until a later session, when the conflict is . . . lukewarm. Then the form of the interpretation would be: "Do you remember last week when you were so upset and (and a reminder is given). I think perhaps you were feeling (and an interpretation is given)." The aim is to make the interpretation usable by the patient, who must have adequate controls to receive it.

Spacing and Length of Appointments

Supportive psychotherapy may consist of a single interview or of sessions spread over a lifetime. As already indicated, acute disturbance may require only a few sessions. A common practice often referred to as spacing and spanning is used when a more extended period of treatment is necessary. This practice consists of regularly scheduled weekly or twice weekly appointments at the outset, subsequently—after a few weeks or a few months—reduced to once every other week and then perhaps once a month or even every other month and finally "prn" (only when the patient calls and expresses the need for an appointment).

In terms of the length of each appointment, the standard 45- or 50-minute "hour" often gives way to a regularly scheduled

30-minute session. In some instances the length of the sessions may vary, depending on what seems optimal for the patient and what is feasible within the therapist's schedule.

Appointments spaced at weekly to monthly intervals and even as brief as 30 minutes may be more meaningful to the patient than the therapist might suspect. This is illustrated by the patient described in Chapter 8 who occasionally needed a "refill."

Short-Term Supportive Psychotherapy

In Chapter 11 we discussed time-limited insight-oriented psychotherapy. A time limit was placed on the psychotherapy as a technique which had as its purposes 1) to increase motivation, 2) to provoke anxiety (to be used in a constructive manner), and 3) to direct a focus on separation and loss issues.

Time-limited techniques may also be indicated with supportive psychotherapy but are used in somewhat different situations and often for different reasons. As a general rule, with supportive psychotherapy the objective is to restore the emotional equilibrium as quickly as possible. With brief supportive psychotherapy, unlike with insight-oriented psychotherapy, new issues would not be raised, but rather patients would be helped to "heal over" areas of discomfort as quickly as possible.

The major indications for short-term supportive psychotherapy are 1) adjustment reactions to acute situational problems that will resolve with minimal interventions and support; 2) persons for whom more prolonged therapy is likely to promote undesired regression or dependency; or 3) situations, such as acute grief, in which limiting therapy emphasizes healthy recuperative processes rather than psychopathology.

Although the recommendation to limit treatment to a few sessions is usually perceived by patients as an indication that a favorable outcome is anticipated, there are some who react as though they are being pushed away. One patient made this clear by speaking of neighbors who would have little to do with her because she had formerly been a drug user. The therapist, in responding, merely stated that the time limit had been selected for therapeutic reasons and not because of her past transgressions.

Therapeutic techniques for brief supportive psychotherapy are essentially the same as for other forms of supportive psychotherapy. One component of such interventions is the use of suggestion in conjunction with proposed brief treatment (for example, "I know that this problem is something that you will be able to master and therefore I recommend that we plan on meeting for only three or four sessions"). Advice and recommendations may be made along with the implication that resolution of the acute difficulty is to be anticipated. Termination may need to be more tentative with brief supportive psychotherapy because the goal is symptom relief rather than "cure" of the underlying problem.

In long-term (open-ended) therapy of grief reactions, the patient faces an ever-present threat of termination and loss of the therapist. This situation can be circumvented to an extent by using a time-limited approach, as described in the next case example.

Mrs. T, a 30-year-old married dependent wife of a military officer, sought help on advice she received from her son's school. The child had much difficulty in separating himself from Mrs. T in the morning when she took him to school. The story quickly emerged that a sibling had been hit by an automobile and killed the previous year. The child who died had suffered from chronic renal disease and was mildly mentally retarded. The mother poignantly talked about the funeral and described how the child had been buried in his favorite clothes, a cowboy outfit complete with boots.

It seemed apparent that the mother was clinging to her healthy child. She was encouraged to grieve more openly and advised that her living child's separation anxiety was a result of her behavior. She was also advised to seek social contacts (e.g., an officers' wives group) outside the home.

A follow-up telephone call from Mrs. T six weeks later indicated that her son had resumed his normal behavior and that she felt much more comfortable. The supportive components of this interaction were acceptance of the patient's grief as a normal process, education (interpretation) as to the nature of her relationship with her living son, and advice on how to shift her dependent needs from the child to a more adult activity.

Supportive techniques can at times be effective in remarkably brief therapy. In the case just cited, treatment consisted of a single hour. The following case required additional time.

Mrs. G, a 63-year-old widow, was referred to a psychiatry clinic by an internist who found no organic pathology to account for her anorexia, weight loss, insomnia, anergy, anhedonia, and crying spells. For her "depression" he prescribed amitriptyline (25 mg hs). Because of her fear of medicines—she had only taken one aspirin in her life—she took one pill and then discarded the rest.

Three months before her first appointment with a psychiatrist, Mrs. G found, upon awakening, that her husband of 43 years had died in his sleep. She told of their close relationship and characterized their pattern as that of "stay-at-homers." Their social contacts had been limited to get-togethers with their two daughters, their daughters' husbands, and their two granddaughters.

While with her daughters or granddaughters, Mrs. G ate and slept well and her other symptoms largely abated. One month after her husband's death her symptoms became much more troublesome when her four-year-old granddaughter, for whom she provided day care, was taken from her and placed in an organized child care program.

The diagnosis was grief reaction in a person who was depressed only when she was alone. Treatment consisted of catharsis and support with the understanding that there would be six 30-minute sessions. Mrs. G was encouraged to mourn her loss. (Her family had tried to keep her from crying.)

It was unfortunate that there were so few persons in Mrs. G's circle. To remedy the situation, and this seemed to be the crucial matter, recommendations were made 1) that Mrs. G move to a setting where there would be the opportunity for companionship, 2) that she explore the possibility of joining a group for the elderly, and 3) that she find employment as a baby sitter (finances were a matter of concern). In other words, she was encouraged to take those steps that would reduce time spent alone.

Two days before Mrs. G's scheduled fifth appointment, she called the therapist to state that she was doing so well that she did not think she needed to come in again. She mentioned that her daughter was letting her do the family laundry once more (a task that made her feel useful) and her granddaughter was spending weekends with her (an arrangement that kept her from feeling lonely). Moreover, her family no longer tried to stop her from grieving. (She had occasional crying spells.)

It seemed evident that Mrs. G's family, with perhaps the best of intentions, had tried to relieve the patient of anything that might be burdensome or upsetting. In doing so they increased the time she spent alone, deprived her of tasks that made her feel useful, and encouraged her to suppress her tears and thereby interfered with the mourning process. When the family perceived that the therapist's approach was in the opposite direction, they reversed their course, with salutary results.

Mrs. G informed the therapist that she had been asked to do some baby sitting and she thought she would take the job. Finally she ended the conversation by saying that the doctor had been of more help to her than he would ever know.

Management

At the more extreme end of the continuum of supportive psychotherapy is management. Management consists of activity on the part of the therapist, usually in the form of advice, persuasion, direction, or manipulation. It may be presented like a prescription with the assumption that the patient will take it as instructed. By reducing pressure the expectation is that discomfort or distress will be relieved.

Sim (1981) commented that in most textbooks of psychiatry there is adequate emphasis on treatment but insufficient emphasis on management. It might be argued that management is a type of treatment, but however it is classified it does not receive sufficient attention.

The following clinical vignette illustrates management technique.

Mrs. B, a 28-year-old woman who had been married for seven years, felt trapped. She had three children, ages four years, two years, and nine months, all by cesarian section. Following the second delivery she developed hypocalcemia and tachycardia and thought she was dying. During her third pregnancy, the only one not planned, she felt extremely anxious. Shortly after the birth of the third child, her husband was transferred and consequently they moved away from family and friends. She found herself housebound because there was little money for sitters, and it was difficult getting around with three little children. As she explained, she could manage two but not three; she only had two hands.

Mr. B was described as a good husband and father. When he was at home he spent much time with the children. Instead of availing herself of the opportunity then to go out, Mrs. B regarded this time as "family time" and spent it with her husband and children. She felt it was her duty to remain at home to care for her children—to be a 24-hour-a-day mother.

Although Mrs. B was anxious and mildly depressed, it seemed appropriate to address her social situation first. Accordingly, practical advice was given in the form of a prescription. She was told that no woman could perform efficiently as a mother unless she reserved sufficient time for her own needs. She was instructed to spend time away from home while her husband looked after the children. It was also declared essential that she and her husband spend at least one evening a week away from home by themselves or with adult company. When seen a month later, Mrs. B stated that she had "mostly" recovered. Only occasionally did she wonder if she would be up to tasks, but her doubts quickly subsided. Chores that had seemed almost insurmountable were easy once again. She had taken up a hobby and spent considerable time shopping. She went out while her husband was at home, and they "dated" at least once a week.

At a six-month follow-up, the improvement had been sustained. Relieving the stressful social situation, in considerable measure self-imposed, resulted in the reestablishment of Mrs. B's emotional equilibrium.

Summary

Supportive psychotherapy includes a wide range of technical interventions that are based on a psychodynamic formulation that takes into account the patient's strengths and weaknesses (ego functions and deficits) and their interaction with current stresses. Treatment strategies may include, at one end of the continuum, supportive interpretations and, at the other extreme, direct environmental manipulation (management).

When maximally effective, supportive psychotherapy utilizes specific interventions based on a well-defined treatment plan. The degree of direct intervention (e.g., provision of advice) is determined by the immediate needs of the patient and his or her current levels of functioning.

13

Psychotherapy Combined with or Augmented by Pharmacotherapy

At present the combination of psychotherapy and pharmacotherapy is well accepted. Such was not always the case. For a time in the past both psychotherapists and psychopharmacologists were reluctant to mix their preferred mode of treatment with the other therapeutic intervention. The reasons for this reluctance have been clearly outlined in the monograph of the Group for the Advancement of Psychiatry (1975) entitled *Pharmacotherapy and Psychotherapy: Paradoxes, Problems, and Progress.* It is not that the problems created by combined therapy can be dismissed as invalid (they are valid!), but rather that the advantages of combined therapy outweigh the disadvantages.

For psychotherapists to maximize the effects of their therapeutic endeavors, it is necessary for them to know the potential advantages as well as the potential disadvantages of the concurrent use of psychotropic medication. Because the indications for, and therapeutic benefits of, psychotropic medication are well described elsewhere, the efficacy of such agents will merely be acknowledged here. Instead, we will focus on the ways in which the concurrent use of psychotropic medications might influence the process of psychotherapy.

Potential Effects of Pharmacotherapy on Psychotherapy

Potential Beneficial Effects

The use of psychopharmacological agents might render patients more accessible for psychotherapy by reducing their discomfort sufficiently to enable them to communicate better and to work more constructively. For example, medication may decrease or eliminate intrusive psychotic ideation and alleviate disabling depression or crippling anxiety and thereby improve cognitive function and memory, reduce distractibility, and promote attention and concentration. Thus, medication may make it possible for patients to engage in psychotherapy who otherwise would find it impossible.

In addressing this issue, Hollender (1965) made the following statement:

> Any concern that tranquilizers, commonly used in office practice, might interfere with psychotherapy has been dispelled by clinical experience. While they do relieve anxiety to an extent, they do not resolve problems. Consequently, motivation remains essentially unimpaired. In fact, if anxiety is severe, palliation may make it easier for the patient to take a problem-oriented approach.

Medication has helped to remove some of the stigma attached to psychiatric illness by identifying it more with the medical-disease model. Thus, the prescription of medication may serve as a vehicle through which patients can seek psychotherapeutic help.

Potential Negative Effects

Many psychiatrists contended that the use of psychotropic medication would have an adverse effect on their relationship with patients. Part of the concern was that the act of prescribing would promote an authoritarian stance on the part of the physician and encourage patients to become more dependent. It was hypothesized that the introduction of medication would initiate or augment countertransference and transference processes and hinder the development of insight. There also was concern that medication might reduce anxiety and relieve other symptoms to such an extent that patients might discontinue psychotherapy. The possibility of "state-learning" was raised. In other words, new information learned under a drug-induced state would be readily available only when the patient was in that particular "state." Yet another concern was that the patient for whom medication was prescribed might experience a loss of self-esteem. This would be particularly likely to occur in patients from a subculture in which a high value is placed on psychotherapy and the use of medication is a "second-class" treatment (Sabshin and Ramot 1956).

Possible Effect of Psychotherapy on Pharmacotherapy

Some pharmacotherapists liken psychotropic drug treatment to the use of certain pharmaceuticals in general medicine. For example, for some disorders a specific psychotropic medication may be viewed as a replacement of a needed metabolite or hormone, much like insulin for diabetes mellitus. With this model, psychotherapy may be viewed as unnecessary or irrelevant. A second argument is that psychotherapy may have a deleterious effect because probing and uncovering defenses may activate anxiety and thereby undercut the therapeutic effectiveness of the drug.

In terms of a positive effect of psychotherapy combined with pharmacotherapy, the approach to panic attacks is an example. After effective treatment with a tricyclic antidepressant (usually imipramine), patients may need psychotherapy to unlearn the anticipatory anxiety and phobic reactions that had developed to cope with the fear of unpredictable panic attacks.

Integration of Pharmacotherapy with Psychotherapy

Karasu (1982) proposed an integrative model for the combination of psychotherapy and medications. He contended that what medication has to offer is often different from what psychotherapy has to offer. Thus, the two treatment approaches, rather than being mutually exclusive, may at times have a synergistic effect. Karasu suggested that medications are most useful for "state" disorders (e.g., depression, anxiety) when symptom relief is the major goal and the disorder is severe, time-limited, and of biological origin. An intervention of this type is often indicated early in treatment and may facilitate access to the patient. Psychotherapy is indicated for "trait" problems which are of long duration, less severe, and interfere primarily with social and interpersonal adjustment.

The following two cases illustrate an integrated approach to psychotherapy and pharmacotherapy. Although they do not necessarily follow the time sequence suggested above, they do demonstrate the complexity of the interactions of the biological and psychodynamic aspects of illness.

A 32-year-old married woman sought psychotherapy because of persistent symptoms of agoraphobia associated with panic attacks. A variety of psychotropic medications prescribed by her internist had all failed to relieve her symptoms. Her history provided prominent evidence of conflicts over autonomy in relationship to a domineering mother, an identification with a passive father who had a history of recurrent major depressions, and ambivalence toward an easy-going, unambitious husband. Psychotherapy provided new insights into these relationships but no relief of symptoms. The addition of phenelzine to her treatment resulted in symptomatic improvement. But more dramatic were the changes in her interpersonal relationships as she became more independent and assertive. In retrospect, the agoraphobia and conflicts over autonomy had acted synergistically to maintain her dependent position. With relief of the panic attacks and agoraphobia, she was able to utilize her new-found insights and effect changes in her life. The combination of an effective medication and insight-oriented psychotherapy created the opportunity for change that neither therapeutic modality alone could have produced.

A 35-year-old single woman attorney presented with chronic depression. Her life-style had been that of a "workaholic," and as such she was exploited by her law firm. Nortriptyline was prescribed after her second visit, and the dosage was gradually increased over several weeks. A pattern emerged in which she would start to feel much better, reduce the dose herself, have a recurrence of symptoms, and then reluctantly increase the dose at the therapist's urging until she felt better, at which point she would again reduce the dose. This self-defeating behavior was puzzling to the psychiatric resident treating the patient until the psychodynamic picture was elucidated. Unconsciously she did not believe that she deserved to feel better, and therefore, paradoxically, she undercut effective treatment. Further, when she felt less depressed, conflicted and uncomfortable sexual and assertive feelings began to emerge.

Although this patient had a medically treatable biological depression, such treatment could not be effectively instituted until she was treated with insight-oriented psychotherapy. The ultimate successful outcome depended on the integrated use of psychotherapy and medication.

The Symbolism of Medication

Even for the most intelligent, sophisticated dyad of patient and therapist, the prescription of medication may be attended by considerable symbolism and evoke irrational emotions and expectations in both halves of the dyad. The physician should have an understanding of the patient's expectations, the potential meanings of the medication, and an awareness of how prescribing or withholding a medication may be used inappropriately to act out feelings.

Medication provokes both the conscious and unconscious reactions associated with magical potions. Traditionally, medication is a substance *prescribed* by a physician (read also as the "omnipotent magician") to create a beneficial and new effect on the passive recipient (the patient). The power of this act can hardly be overestimated. The "placebo effect" has been demonstrated to produce physiological changes in subjects, an effect *not* related to traits such as suggestibility, hysteria, low education, or defective intelligence. Similarly, in addition to potent beneficial action, placebos may produce adverse side effects (Wolf and Pinsky 1954). Thus, the magical potion may be unconsciously regarded as good magic or as potentially powerful and destructive magic.

A medication given to a patient may serve as an extension of the physician. In other words, when patients receive the physician's medication and leave the office, a part of the physician goes with them. A specific medication may become strongly identified with either positive or negative feelings toward a particular physician. This is clearly demonstrated in clinics where psychiatric residents rotate as therapists for patients. In such a setting the importance of the drugs prescribed by a physician with whom the patient has a warm and affectionate relationship can be observed. The prescription and the taking of the medication represent a continuation of that good relationship.

If a new resident feels threatened by the relationship the patient had with the previous resident, one of the first "therapeutic" acts may be discontinuing the medication previously prescribed and substituting something new. Such behavior, of course, usually stems from unconscious competition. The patient, who is likely to resent the intrusion into the old relationship, may develop an adverse reaction to the new medication.

Based on the symbolism involved, it can be surmised that some statements made by a patient about a particular medication, either positive or negative, may be a reflection of the quality of the relationship between the patient and physician. For example, a young woman admitted to the hospital after taking an overdose of a psychotropic medication, when asked by her therapist if she had used the medication he had prescribed in the overdose, responded, "No. I would never have overdosed on the medicine that *you* prescribed!"

The symbolism of medication is important to the physician as well as the patient. A prescription may be regarded as a "gift" and therefore a positive act. On occasion, however, giving medication may be regarded as "punishment" and used to express anger. An example is that of the frustrated and angry physician who increases the dosage of a phenothiazine and insists that it be given intramuscularly.

The prescription of a drug may create the aura of an authoritarian relationship, and patients may regard taking it as permission to accept a more dependent role. In a sense, too, the prescription may be regarded as a magical potion given by a physician who is omnipotent and omniscient. Failure to achieve the desired result places the onus on the physician for being less powerful than had been imagined and thus withholding a potential bounty from the patient. This situation is frequently seen in pain clinics, where the patient typically demands that the physician take responsibility for the relief of pain.

Psychotropic Medications in Insight-Oriented Psychotherapy

At one time many classical psychoanalysts were reluctant to use medication in association with insight-oriented psychotherapy. When it was deemed absolutely necessary, they might insist that the medication be prescribed by another physician or by an "administrative psychiatrist" rather than prescribe it themselves. It must be recognized, however, that there are constitutional and genetic differences in temperament and predisposition to such disorders as bipolar affective disorder and panic attacks that require a biological approach. Furthermore, some life experiences are so overwhelming emotionally that they leave an indelible mark that affects the individual's capacity to respond to certain situations. Such adverse experiences may include, but are not limited to, incarceration in a concentration camp (Rappaport 1968), repetitive physical and emotional abuse during childhood, and the death of a parent early in childhood.

The pragmatic therapist must accept the fact that insight does not alleviate some symptoms and that the patient must learn to accept certain aspects of psychic functioning as "givens." While some symptoms cannot be changed, others can be altered only by direct physical intervention, such as with a medication. The patient may have more difficulty than the therapist in accepting this limitation.

One of the objectives of insight-oriented psychotherapy is to help patients recognize their innate physical and psychological characteristics and learn how these interacted with environmental events to produce different psychological constellations and symptoms. Dysphoric feelings may result from endogenous affective disorders and a high degree of emotional lability (mood reactivity). Panic attacks and anxiety may be generated or more intensely experienced when there is hypersensitivity produced by central nervous system abnormalities. And, in addition, one of the more prized aspects of self, thinking, may be disordered as a result of schizophrenia, now generally considered to be primarily due to brain dysfunction rather than psychogenic influences. The foregoing emphasizes the necessity of recognizing that the patient's ego is continuously mediating between instinctual forces and affectual states generated internally and the milieu externally. These endogenous states are as different for each individual as their life experiences.

The following vignette reported by Cooper (1985) illustrates one type of combined therapy.

> *As the analysis of a woman progressed, she became calmer, was able to pursue her work successfully, began to develop a much higher level of self-esteem, and had somewhat better relationships with men. Despite these improvements, she would episodically revert to the symptoms with which she had entered treatment: a mixed depressive-anxious state with feelings of shame and worthlessness, terrified that she would be rejected.*
>
> *Two years after termination the patient called her analyst in a state of mixed depression and panic, the kind of feeling with which she had entered analysis. It occurred to the analyst that she might be describing a recurrent biologic dysregulation and that a search for further psychological content might not be productive. That thought had also occurred to her. Despite much trepidation, she agreed to a trial of imipramine. She responded well to the medication despite side effects and stated that she felt relieved and*

> *reorganized and had the sense that an outside intrusion into her life, the severe anxiety, had been alleviated. She had the feeling that in some way she was more in control of herself than she had ever been.*
>
> *This woman later decided to return for further psychotherapy to deal with conflictual aspects of her life that had not been successfully analyzed while anxiety and mood dysregulation were, perhaps independently, dominating her ongoing psychological life.*

Cooper (1985) elegantly described the ways in which new information concerning neurobiology may be incorporated in the psychological treatment of patients. He noted that with our greater understanding of anxiety, the analyst (therapist) is confronted with the need to determine what portion of a patient's anxiety is relatively nonpsychological (physiological in etiology) and what portion is due to psychic conflicts. He indicated that anxiety and mood dysregulation, constitutional in origin, might dominate a patient's ongoing psychological life. Control of this discomfort by medication may enhance self-esteem and the capacity to focus effectively on content-related psychodynamic issues. He pointed out that, at least with one patient, the endogenously generated affective symptoms were used "masochistically as proof that she was an innocent victim of endless emotional pain."

What is implied by the foregoing discussion is the need for the therapist to view a patient simultaneously from the perspective of both the biological substrata and psychological operations. Patients employ defensive mechanisms to cope with emotional states internally generated as well as those occurring in response to external events.

Prescribing Medication

The physician who prescribes medication within an insight-oriented psychotherapy must avoid an authoritarian stance. Instead, and consistent with the physician-patient model of mutual participation, the physician should explain to the patient why medication is indicated, how it is likely to be effective, and both its potential advantages and disadvantages. Because the goal is to achieve a greater understanding, both psychologically and physiologically, the meaning of the medication (including its transferential aspects) needs to be discussed fully. Thus, unlike many situations in supportive psychotherapy, there should be no effort to amplify the placebo effect.

The therapist who prescribes medication during insight-oriented psychotherapy needs to be a knowledgeable psychopharmacologist in order to determine if what the patient reports in response to the medication is physiological or if it is a symbolic communication. Medication, when appropriately used along with insight-oriented psychotherapy, should be integrated into the patient's increasingly greater understanding of how he or she operates physiologically as well as psychologically and how a pharmacological agent affects both. This is a difficult but intellectually stimulating task.

Selecting the appropriate time to start a medication is important. If it is anticipated that insight-oriented psychotherapy will be recommended, medication is seldom started during the evaluation phase. To prescribe a medication before the therapeutic alliance is well established is likely to provoke complex transference issues that may be difficult to unravel. Further, without a clear knowledge of the patient's usual "steady-state," it may be difficult to know whether changes in symptoms and functioning are due to the medication or to other factors. For example, most patients experience a significant reduction in their perception of acute stress after the first few visits to the therapist. There are many psychological reasons for this, and if a drug is prescribed during this period, it may erroneously be regarded as the effective therapeutic agent.

Indications for the Use of Medication

The need for pharmacotherapy during insight-oriented psychotherapy often involves a difficult and subtle decision. The patients are usually not severely disabled because if they were another form of treatment would have been recommended. A general statement might be that psychotropic medication has a role when, in the opinion of both therapist and patient, the symptoms create a disruption in the patient's life, are not likely to be resolved by further understanding of their etiology, and are characteristically responsive to a specific pharmacological intervention (e.g., imipramine for panic attacks). The following case is illustrative.

> *A middle-aged businessman sought treatment for severe separation anxiety most prominent when it was necessary to make business trips away from home. The cause of his anxiety seemed fairly transparent. He had suffered multiple losses during childhood, including the death of his mother,*

deportation from his home in Hungary, and finally an anxiety-provoking emigration to the United States where he had to learn English before pursuing a business career. He worked cooperatively in psychotherapy and believed that he functioned better and with greater overall psychological comfort, but he continued to experience the uncomfortable symptoms of separation anxiety. Given the degree of early trauma, further insight or working-through were not likely to have an impact upon the symptom. The prescription of an anxiolytic drug for situational use proved effective and, because the decision was reached by mutual agreement, such use was not regarded with guilt for having "copped out."

At times, insight-oriented psychotherapy is used to treat conflicts that initially appear to be psychogenic but later appear to be primarily endogenous in nature. For these patients, medications may play a major role. It is also possible, as illustrated by the following case history, for an endogenous disorder (in this instance a major depression) to develop during the course of psychotherapy.

A middle-aged professional man sought treatment because of symptoms of anxiety and fear of public speaking. Initially psychotherapy revolved around issues related to his unfulfilled dependency wishes and feelings of being in competition with his young wife, who was aggressively successful in her career. The emergence during therapy of transitory sexual difficulties was interpreted as reflecting concerns about masculinity engendered by his competitive wife. Later, however, the development of persistent insomnia led to the suspicion of a major depression. A treatment plan that included prescription of a monoamine oxidase inhibitor (the patient had been unresponsive to a trial of tricyclic antidepressants at an earlier time in his life) was recommended and agreed on. This treatment proved effective and within several weeks the patient recognized that he was his "usual self" and able once again to participate in insight-oriented psychotherapy.

Relative Contraindications for Medication

To a large extent the reasons not to use medication are the obverse of the indications. Medication should not be used to treat minor or transitory periods of dysphoria. At our current level of understanding, they have little place in the treatment of character disorders, and they should not be used for nonspecific purposes when the target symptoms are poorly defined. The use of medication is particularly ill advised when it may add another complicating variable to an already complex and difficult crisis in psychotherapy.

Potential Problems of Combined Therapy

The concurrent use of medication and psychotherapy may create technical problems that need continuous monitoring. Some areas of potential difficulty are listed below.

Medication may be used as a resistance and divert attention from the task of psychotherapy. When medication is prescribed, some time must be devoted to inquiring about both beneficial and adverse reactions. Thus, attention may be diverted from the major issues being discussed in psychotherapy. If the psychodynamic issues make either party uncomfortable, there is the danger that concern about or attention to the somatic aspects of treatment may be used to interfere with psychotherapy. Both physician and patient should guard against the tendency to become preoccupied with somatic issues at times of difficulty or discomfort and acknowledge openly this form of resistance when it occurs. There is also the possibility that *displacement* may occur because it may be easier to discuss various aspects of physiological function, such as sexuality, in terms of the medication's effect than in terms of the intrapsychic focus and affect.

Medication can serve as a scapegoat (displacement) for issues within the therapy situation. This particular problem is, of course, similar to the use of medication as a resistance. In this instance the medication can be the focus of attention by either the physician, or the patient, or both. Continued dysphoric affect, failure to progress in therapy, setbacks, and a variety of somatic complaints may all be blamed on medication or "drug failure" rather than on failure of psychotherapy.

> *A woman repetitively sought psychotherapy supposedly to deal with depression related to her husband's infidelity. Successively, several therapists tried antidepressant medication. Each course of treatment had been accompanied by a transient improvement, only to be followed by a relapse and anger directed at the medication and at the physicians*

who had failed her, as her husband had. Therapy was successful when her therapist was able to confront her with her anger and interpret the "drug failures" as the patient's use of depression to punish her husband.

Overeagerness to prescribe may result from the physician's feelings of inadequacy or failure as a psychotherapist. This problem is seen principally under two circumstances. The first is the frustration that a therapist feels when a patient's symptoms are not responding to psychotherapy. The compelling feeling then may be that one must do something for the patient. The patient's continued dysphoria may elicit such discomfort in the therapist that he or she begins to feel like a failure and starts to search for an alternative approach that will bring success. At such times medication may be indicated, but more often the prescriptions are written impulsively and are not targeted for symptoms that are known to be responsive to a specific medication.

A second commonly seen phenomenon is the therapist who, uncertain of skills and dubious of the efficacy of psychotherapy in the best of circumstances, is quick to prescribe drugs to gain a feeling of doing something for the patient. This happens when the therapist is a physician and therefore accustomed to ending office visits with the "gift" of a prescription.

Some therapists fail to prescribe medication when indicated because of narcissism or grandiosity in regard to psychotherapy skills. For these therapists a prescription represents a personal failure. This attitude is often associated with a preconception that specific psychodynamics are the etiological basis for most psychiatric disorders. Recently such an attitude has become less common.

Medication may represent a venue for acting-out by either the patient or the physician. It is not unusual for patients, consciously or unconsciously, to view the prescription of medication as a gift or as something that is due them. In an attempt to prove that they are loved, patients may continuously try to obtain medication by manipulating the physician. Such manipulations may also reflect a low self-esteem with an effort to feel more powerful by "putting one over" on the physician. Thus, medication may take on the quality of currency in interpersonal transactions.

Besides the "game" played in an effort to obtain prescriptions, patients may also fail to take drugs as prescribed. Compliance is a complex issue determined by multiple factors (Docherty and Fiester 1985). One factor, reflective of the psychotherapeutic relationship, is seen in patients who fail to take medications when they are angry at the physician, as if to punish him or her.

Patients are not the only guilty parties in potential nonmedical use (or nonuse) of medication. Physicians may fail to prescribe needed medication when they are angry or bored with patients. The converse is that at times of anger or frustration, the therapist may prescribe medication that is not required.

Medication and Supportive Psychotherapy

With supportive psychotherapy the repression of anxiety and other dysphoric affects is emphasized, and existing ego defense mechanisms are supported. Little attention is focused on the acquisition of insight by the patient, and the transference is seldom interpreted. Psychotropic medications are used frequently and in such a manner as to take advantage of the positive transference.

To be most effective, medication must be used within the confines of the patients' own psychological view of the world and in ways that are ego-syntonic. The following clinical note is an example.

> *A young woman who had recently given birth to her first child presented with the symptom of anxiety severe enough to disrupt her capacity to care for the child. Other information of importance was that she had limited financial resources for extended insight-oriented psychotherapy and was not psychologically minded. The psychodynamic assessment indicated that she was experiencing "signal anxiety" in response to the threatened emergence of her own angry impulses toward her child, who was demanding the dependent care for which she herself longed so desperately.*
>
> *However, the issue was conflicted because the child was planned and strongly desired, and also had cemented a generally positive relationship for the patient with her husband. The therapist, after careful consideration, prescribed a benzodiazepine for anxiety and explained that because of the medication it would be necessary for her to discontinue breast-feeding. She was praised for the excellent care she was providing her infant, and the therapist's comments emphasized the positive relationship she had with her husband.*

Within two to three days there was a marked decrease in the patient's anxiety. She experienced a rise in self-esteem, and her ability to function as a mother and wife returned. Later both the anxiolytic medication and psychotherapy were discontinued without a recurrence of symptoms.

Within the supportive psychotherapy model the approach to this woman focused on 1) the prescription on a transient basis of a benzodiazepine that reduced her anxiety so that she could sleep and provide effective care for her infant, and 2) emphasis of the sense of accomplishment she received from caring for her child and from the positive relationship she had with her husband. It is possible that the medication also provided an ego-syntonic excuse to discontinue breast-feeding. However, this issue was never explored with her.

The following case note illustrates another use of medication within a supportive framework.

A woman in her late fifties with multiple somatic symptoms suggestive of an endogenous depression had resisted her internist's suggestions that she take tricyclic antidepressant medication. Consciously she feared that it would control her but, more importantly, unconsciously she felt she did not deserve it. At her internist's insistence she finally accepted a referral for a psychiatric consultation. The psychiatrist, who detected underlying masochistic personality traits in association with the major depression, emphasized that although the antidepressant medication would be effective, it also would cause many unpleasant side effects such as dryness of the mouth, sedation, and constipation. It was explained to her that she would have to endure these unpleasant symptoms in order to gain some beneficial relief. The idea that the patient would not get something for nothing was consistent with her need to suffer, and taking the prescribed medication then became more ego-syntonic. As she became less depressed the therapist was able, in supportive psychotherapy, to help her see that self-sacrificing for her adult son and daughter had only perpetuated their immaturity. She was encouraged to direct her need to serve others in a more constructive manner—namely, volunteer work at a local convalescent hospital. The patient's unconscious rage at her husband and son and daughter and her need to atone for it through masochistic behavior was not interpreted to her.

With many supportive psychotherapy patients who require ongoing psychotropic medication, positive feelings between the therapist and the patient help to facilitate compliance. A patient with a history of a bipolar affective disorder who requires lithium will be more likely to continue taking the medication as prescribed if there are warm feelings toward the physician who prescribed it. As mentioned previously, the medication then becomes valued as a part of the positive relationship. In such an ongoing relationship, the physician will usually elect not to deal in an insightful way with the patient's feelings toward him or her. Instead, education as to the nature of the medication, its indications, potential side effects, and positive beneficial action may become the central focus of the therapeutic relationship. In this form of therapy the physician would be disinclined to interpret the unconscious symbolic meanings of the medication.

Summary

The development of effective psychotropic medication has been an important addition to the psychiatrist's armamentarium. With the availability of medication, treatment has become more complex, particularly when the two therapeutic modalities are combined. However, as long as the therapist is aware of the potential complications and prescribes judiciously, the net therapeutic benefit can be very great.

14

Problem Situations and Difficult Patients

In this chapter we will first discuss practical issues that, unless handled thoughtfully, may lead to problems. Then we will turn our attention to several personality patterns that have special impact on the therapist-patient relationship.

Problem Situations

Silences

In social situations, a good host and hostess will see to it that their guests do not have to face awkward, tension-producing periods of silence. Talking may serve to conceal feelings that might be disturbing or embarrassing.

In treatment situations, letting periods of silence continue may be appropriate or inappropriate. When appropriate, the therapist should be able to tolerate these periods. Because such behavior runs counter to a previously learned pattern, it calls for unlearning.

As previously stated (see Chapter 7), prolonged periods of silence may be poorly tolerated by patients, especially during the early phase of treatment. Silence is likely to have the greatest impact on persons raised in homes in which silence was used as a form of severe punishment. For them, during the evaluation period or early phase of treatment, therapists are well advised to make some comments, however brief and bland, to relieve the mounting tension. A question such as "What are you thinking?" may serve the purpose.

In supportive psychotherapy, if silences are anxiety-producing, an effort should be made to eliminate them.

With prolonged silences during insight-oriented psychotherapy, interventions (comments and interpretations) should be directed toward the silence itself in an effort to understand its meaning within the therapeutic process. As Sullivan (1954) stated, "Anyone who proceeds without consideration for the disjunctive power of anxiety in human relationships will never learn interviewing."

Last-Minute Spurts

What should the therapist do if a patient brings up a new and important topic just minutes before the end of the hour? Although the therapist need not be so inflexible that he or she will not permit the patient occasionally to run five or 10 minutes over, especially if the topic is sensitive and perhaps painful, this should not become a frequent occurrence.

A different type of situation is created when a patient, near the end of an hour, inquires if it would be possible for him to have two appointments a week instead of one—an important question but not a pressing one. Rather than give a hurried and, at best, a partial answer, it is better to defer the answer. Accordingly, the therapist informs the patient that the issue merits more careful scrutiny and consideration than would be possible in the time remaining in the present hour, and therefore it would be better to consider it at the next hour or at a later date.

Note-Taking and Recordings

Note-taking may place a barrier between the therapist and patient, thereby interfering with a free and natural interchange. It is true, however, that most patients in a short time become accustomed to note-taking. Then, if the therapist writes less or stops writing altogether, the patient is likely to conclude that the therapist has lost interest. The fact that patients become accustomed to note-taking should not be regarded as confirmation of its desirability; undesirable conditions may be tolerated or accepted in the interest of maintaining a relationship that is, or seems to be, useful.

Audiotape recordings have sometimes been used in the place of note-taking. The use of the tape recorder eliminates the problems of divided attention and selective reporting. But there is one serious disadvantage: the invasion of privacy. Statements made by patients in their own voice can be potentially more damaging than statements that are only imputed to them. The barrier created in this manner may be insurmountable for very suspicious and guarded patients. Others, who are less fearful and cautious, may tolerate the procedure if they receive assurance that the tapes will be available only to the therapist and perhaps a supervisor or consultant. But how can they be certain? Usually to adjust to the recording of interviews patients must accept the therapist's assurance, be more circumspect in what they say, or push the matter out of their mind. In one of these ways, or perhaps some other, patients make their peace and pay a price for the help they receive.

In recent years videotape recordings of sessions may be used for supervision. Their advantage for educational purposes is obvious, but their use has the potential for an even greater invasion of privacy than audiotapes. For some patients the presence of a camera may be more intrusive than a microphone.

One-way mirrors, with an instructor or students hidden from view, have also been popular with some teaching programs for many years. When this arrangement is used for diagnostic purposes, however, it may be more distracting than having the observers physically present in the room with the patient and the interviewer. With unseen observers many critical or belittling fantasy pictures may be conjured up. Still, in so-called observed psychotherapy the use of the one-way mirror may have some advantages. It is noteworthy that in an ongoing process the patient is likely to adjust and adapt to an awareness of observers more quickly than the therapist. (Of course, the patient is always informed whenever a one-way mirror is used.)

Patients may agree to the recording of sessions but covertly resent being called on to do so. This situation and its management are illustrated by the following clinical example.

> *A 38-year-old woman in treatment by a supervised trainee gave her permission for audiotaping. In subsequent sessions, however, there were more prolonged silences and muffled speech and less discussion of personally important issues. It was pointed out that she had acquiesced to the therapist's request for her permission to record their sessions rather than express her feelings. This reaction was similar to her reaction to her husband—"going with the flow" in a passively noncooperative manner.*

Additional Appointments

Although sessions are not usually added to the number originally agreed upon, provision should be made for exceptions. Occasionally the time between appointments is longer than anxious or distraught patients can tolerate. An extra hour not only makes it possible to come to grips with a problem while feelings are intense, but it also shortens the period of turmoil. An extra appointment also should be scheduled for patients on the brink of a panic reaction or beset by strong suicidal impulses. On the other hand, the therapist should hold the line with patients who would like to turn over their care to someone else and sink further and further into a helpless and dependent state. In these instances the line should be held with a show of kindness that is matched by firmness.

What has been said about appointments also applies to telephone calls. For some patients, an occasional call makes it possible to extend the time between office visits, whereas for other patients who lean too heavily and too often on calls, it may be necessary to restrict the number and length of the calls.

Telephone Calls from the Patient's Spouse, Relatives, or Friends

During the early phase of treatment, a patient's spouse may call seeking information. She may say, "I'm concerned about my husband, and I would like to ask a few questions. Do you have time to talk to me now, or can I make an appointment to see you?" The questions usually pertain to the nature, and especially the seriousness, of the spouse's illness, the treatment to be instituted, and the prognosis.

In terms of medical situations generally, the wife is behaving appropriately. No one would think it unusual if she were to call a family practitioner or internist to inquire about her husband's illness and to learn if she might do something that would be helpful.

How the therapist responds to the wife's call should depend upon the nature of the husband's illness and the type of treatment prescribed. If the approach is supportive psychotherapy, the therapist may wish to see the spouse and accordingly would suggest that she accompany the patient to his next appointment. Concern about suicidal impulses, the handling of medication, and environmental manipulation may dictate the role the wife should play. In supportive psychotherapy, the response to telephone calls may essentially be like the usual response to them in medical practice.

For insight-oriented psychotherapy, special considerations are in order for handling telephone calls. Although the therapist understands that the spouse's call may be an appropriate expression of interest and concern, the therapist should state that because of the nature of the treatment it is not possible to discuss the patient's problems with the spouse. Following a brief explanation, the therapist might state, "I hope you will appreciate why I am not at liberty to discuss your husband's treatment with you." Before ending the call, the therapist should mention, "It would be best if I told your husband that you called and what I said to you." Whether so intended or not, this practice tends to discourage further calls.

In addition to spouses, other close relatives, and friends who call the therapist to seek information, there are those who call to impart information. Again, the therapist's approach should be determined by the nature of the therapy. It may be of great importance to obtain outside information about the patient in supportive psychotherapy. For the patient in insight-oriented psychotherapy, quite the opposite is true. Thus, the would-be informant should be told that providing information would be antithetical to the goals of treatment.

Patients Who Bring or Send Friends or Relatives to a Therapy Session

It is not unusual during the course of some types of psychotherapy for a patient or therapist to suggest that a joint session with a significant other, usually a spouse, be arranged. In these situations it is possible to discuss the goals of such a meeting, anticipate complications, and agree upon how the time will be spent.

Occasionally patients will unexpectedly bring someone with them to an appointment and ask that he or she be permitted to remain for the therapy session. Except in unusual circumstances, requests of this type should be politely but firmly denied and the meaning of bringing the visitor explored during the hour.

The following clinical example illustrates the type of situation created when a patient sends a "visitor."

> *A therapist went to the waiting room to meet his scheduled patient, but found instead a man who introduced himself as the patient's husband. The husband explained that he had been sent so that the therapist could explain to him how he (the husband) could better meet the patient's needs. The therapist spent approximately 15 minutes with the husband and during their brief discussion asked the husband, "Does your wife often do things that make you angry?" Later the therapist became aware that the question was prompted by his own anger at the patient's tendency toward*

manipulation. (Issues of the patient's narcissism and manipulation, as evidenced by this behavior, were later dealt with in her therapy.)

In retrospect a better way of handling this awkward and difficult situation would have been to firmly decline to see the husband, giving no more information than that such a visit would be "inappropriate."

Nonpayment (or Late Payment) of Fees

Most patients recognize their financial obligation and make their payment promptly. For some, however, the payment of fees becomes a battleground. What cannot be expressed in words is expressed in this manner. Some therapists who are uncomfortable in asking for money (this discomfort perhaps representing a subtle devaluation of their services) may permit the accumulation of a substantial debt that increasingly causes tension between them and their patients.

Therapists also devalue their services by acceding to the request to have clinic fees reduced (or eliminated) from the usual schedule. Although at times there may be realistic reasons for such a change, it is necessary to guard against being an accomplice in a patient's manipulations.

Psychotherapy trainees are particularly likely to be reluctant to discuss financial issues and may accede to a reduction or even elimination of the fee schedule. They may devalue their services and feel guilty about charging the patient a fee. However, such a stance also serves to devalue the therapy in the patient's eyes and thereby undercuts the therapeutic process. It is essential that the therapist, whether in a clinic or private practice, remain aware of the payment of fees and address the matter directly if the agreed-to schedule is not maintained.

Telephone Calls from the Patient

It is the therapist's responsibility to be available to respond to emergencies and to accept telephone calls of an appropriate businesslike nature (e.g., canceled appointments because of illness). Some patients attempt to overuse the telephone. The reasons for this include 1) dependency with separation anxiety, 2) an eroticized transference, 3) hostile dependency (with the knowledge that frequent calls can be irritating), and 4) an attempt to extend the time of therapy, often with the fantasy of not having to pay for it.

If a therapist receives multiple telephone calls other than for genuine emergencies, it is possible that there has been a subtle encouragement of dependency. If so, the problem may lie more with the therapist than the patient.

Telephone calls should be discussed during subsequent therapy sessions. If calls persist then it may be necessary to set more structured rules as to frequency. Some therapists, similar to attorneys, charge for telephone calls.

Social Encounters with Patients

Even in large cities therapists are likely to encounter patients at social gatherings. Those patients who do not wish to interact with their therapist will keep their distance. At a cocktail party they will stay on the opposite side of the room. Those who wish to make the most of this chance meeting will join the group that the therapist is with. Most patients, however, will probably merely say hello and wander off. The therapist should keep his or her distance from the patients who have indicated this preference and he or she should be as natural as possible with the others.

Although chance meetings cannot be avoided, planned ones can be. Therefore, it should be understood that therapists will neither extend social invitations to patients nor accept social invitations from them.

Following social encounters, therapists should be on the alert for reactions to them that come forth in the material of the next hour or two. As would be expected, the nature of the response may be largely shaped by matters under consideration at the time.

Gifts

It is mainly at Christmas time that patients come bearing gifts. On the surface this custom-sanctioned act appears to be as innocuous as it is traditional, but as real as the spirit of the season may be it is less than "100 proof." Various motives—some conscious and others unconscious—dilute it, sometimes markedly. Among these motives are bids for special attention, a profound and unreasonable sense of indebtedness, and a feeling that some token is expected or even required.

Gifts are either handmade by the giver or purchased. The personal investment of self in the former is bound to be much greater than in the latter. Some therapists—and we are in the group—would rarely if ever turn down a handmade gift because no matter what explanation is offered this would be a shattering experience for the patient.

A token gift purchased by the patient may be accepted or refused. In either case the motives impelling the patient to give it should be discussed. Usually the motives will be evident in the material of the hour. Very expensive gifts should always be declined.

Therapists who are showered with gifts should take stock and ask, "What message am I sending?" They should wonder if they are being overly nice to their patients and as a result engendering a feeling of obligation. Therapists who receive many gifts should scrutinize their own behavior before looking for their patients' motives.

A special circumstance may exist for therapists and patients in a clinic. Because of low fees, even though patients know that the therapists' salary comes from the clinic, they may feel a sense of indebtedness that is the motive for giving a gift. In this instance the basic factor is situational and accordingly the gift may be accepted without the need to scrutinize the patients' motive or the therapists' part.

Missed Appointments or Tardiness

If an appointment is missed and if an explanation is not forthcoming at the next hour, the therapist should inquire about what happened. Not to do so would suggest that the therapist does not regard the patient and therapy as important. The tone of voice in which the question is asked may be received as an inquiry expressing interest and concern or as a form of chastisement.

If an appointment is missed early in therapy, it may be appropriate for the therapist to call and inquire why. The question might be asked, "I wonder if there was some misunderstanding. I had expected to see you at. . . . " The call might clarify genuine misunderstandings. It may also signify interest and have a salutary effect.

Recurrent missed appointments is cause for exploration and explanation. Is this evidence of a strong resistance? Or is it a nonverbal way of indicating that nothing of sufficient value is gained from coming to an hour to make it worth the extra effort that might be involved? When missing appointments is consistent with the patient's characteristic behavior, this fact should have been noted during the evaluation period and discussed then. The original discussion may need to be repeated during the course of therapy.

Some patients who are chronically late may maintain that they just never try to adhere "compulsively" to a time schedule. The striking fact is that they are almost always exactly the same number of minutes late: five minutes or seven minutes or 10 minutes. In these instances being late may be the expression of rebelliousness in a person who grew up in a strict family where there were very few ways to rebel. Other dynamic patterns may be found responsible for chronic or episodic tardiness. When there is so often a "good reason" for being late, this pattern should be pointed out.

The time lost due to lateness is not usually made up. Only in highly unusual circumstances would it be appropriate to extend a session in response to a patient's lateness.

Difficult Situations Related to the Therapist

At times there are events in the therapist's life that have an impact on psychotherapy; these may be unavoidable. We will discuss two of them but recognize that there are many other possibilities.

The Therapist's Illness

It may be necessary to cancel one or more sessions with a patient because of illness. With more serious illness there may be an extended break in the therapy. In other situations the therapist may have some obvious physical sign of illness or disability, e.g., crutches, a cast, or a visible bandage. Usually a brief statement about the nature of the difficulty will suffice and the patient can continue to work in therapy. The therapist, however, should be on the lookout for the patient's fantasies about his or her injury or illness.

The Therapist's Pregnancy

A therapist's pregnancy creates some unique problems and presents some valuable opportunities in psychotherapy (Nadelson et al. 1974). The pregnant therapist must deal with feelings of increased vulnerability, both physical and emotional. The pregnancy may also exacerbate issues of role identity or dependency in professional relationships. There may also be increased internal difficulty in dealing with patient issues such as abortion.

The therapist's pregnancy may evoke a number of different feelings or fantasies in the patient. Among these are an intensified maternal transference, awareness of the therapist as a sexual person, competition with the baby or the therapist's husband, and separation anxiety due to an anticipated break in therapy. Nadelson et al. (1974) recommended that the pregnancy be dealt with in an open and realistic manner. The result—working on the issues stimulated or intensified by the pregnancy—is likely to be a particularly productive experience.

Difficult Patients

Michels (1977) stated, "Psychotherapy is difficult. Indeed there are many who believe that it is impossible. For the rest of us the impression persists that although it is always problematic, there are certain patients . . . [who] present particular difficulty."

A particular diagnosis in itself may suggest that a patient will be difficult, such as in patients with dysmorphophobia. In thinking of groupings of difficult patients, however, we are likely to think in terms of particular personality traits. Thus, we speak of the seductive patient, the manipulative patient, the dependent patient, and the needful or demanding patient. Other potentially difficult patients are persons who hold a position of power or influence and patients who induce boredom in the therapist.

In the sections that follow, we will describe the more common types of difficult patients encountered in clinical practice.

The Seductive Patient

The classic picture is the sexually seductive, attractive female patient in treatment with a young male therapist. The following discussion will focus on this combination, but first it should be pointed out that seduction efforts can, and often do, take other forms. There are, for instance, women and men who appeal to the therapist's narcissism. Some therapists find it relatively easy to deal with attempts at erotic seduction but find it difficult to withstand appeals to their vanity. There are also male patients who attempt to ingratiate themselves by offering their therapist tips on the stock market or other financially attractive deals. This, in a broad sense, is also an attempt at seduction.

The seductive patient in the classic sense is most likely to have the traits usually associated with the hysterical personality. Subtly, or not so subtly, she may attempt to convert a professional relationship into a social one with erotic overtones. Information may be sought about the therapist's personal interests, late afternoon or evening appointments may be requested, and the therapist's skill may be compared—favorably of course—with those of previous therapists (Hollender and Shevitz 1978).

If a therapist regularly spends more than the usual amount of time with a patient, he should ask himself why. If he finds himself repeatedly thinking or talking about a particular patient, on introspection he may conclude that she fascinates him, and the feeling of fascination (or perhaps even infatuation) should be a clear warning signal.

The seductiveness of the woman with the life-style of the hysterical personality is clearly the coyness or fetching behavior of a little girl. What is really being sought is attention and nurture—mothering. The therapist, like other men, may misread her and assume she is seeking a sexual encounter.

If seductive behavior provides a harmless glow and clearly is within reasonable bounds, nothing need or should be done about it. If it threatens to break out of bounds, there are several options of which doing nothing may be the least desirable. One approach is to point out the behavior and to interpret the meaning of it (i.e., the use of seductiveness in the interest of obtaining attention and nurture). An occasional patient may need to be reminded that it would be more difficult for her to find a competent therapist than a good sexual partner, and therefore it would be wise to hold onto this strictly professional relationship (Lisansky 1976).

The following clinical vignette, originally reported by Halleck (1978), is of interest both from the standpoint of the dynamic pattern presented and the manner in which the seductive behavior was dealt with in treatment.

> *A 22-year-old woman in therapy for problems of mild anxiety and depression became seductive toward her therapist. She talked openly about how she found him sexy. She began to dress in a very appealing manner and made it clear that she would be quite willing to have a love affair with him. The patient had a long history of using her sexual attractiveness to gain control of situations in which she felt insecure. However, after she began a sexual relationship with a man, she would quickly become guilty and depressed. The therapist in this case acknowledged the patient's advances,*

> *said he felt complimented that she found him attractive, but also pointed out that, since both of them were involved in a professional relationship in which she was seeking help for emotional problems, it would be most fruitful to spend their time investigating the purpose or meaning of her seductive behavior.*

With no apparent encouragement from the therapist and in spite of interpretations of the meaning of the seductive behavior, some patients continue actively to express their desire for a sexual relationship. Their behavior may include frequent telephone calls and efforts to learn more about the details of the therapist's personal life, at times going to the extreme of contacting the therapist's friends. Such behavior obviously interferes with the therapeutic process. The therapist may decide to terminate therapy or to insist that the patient see a colleague, in consultation, in an effort to determine if some complicating factors in the therapy have been overlooked by the primary therapist.

The Manipulative Patient

The behavior labeled manipulative is usually a covert bid for special attention, attention that exceeds the limits previously agreed upon. If the therapist focuses on the violation of the agreement rather than the behavior as evidence of psychopathology the relationship in all likelihood, will shift from therapeutic to adversarial. Mackenzie et al. (1978) stated, "The accusation that a patient is manipulative signals the disruption of the helping process." They also pointed out that the term manipulative is associated with anger on the part of the therapist and a sense of the impossibility of his or her task. They continued,

> Its use almost always seems to signal an impending breakdown in the helping process and a shift to an adversary relationship between therapist and patient. It moves the patient into a conceptual space where his demands are no longer legitimate and where his treatment failure becomes "his own fault."

Mackenzie et al. (1978) also stated,

> The initial step toward repairing the therapeutic dyad is to acknowledge that one is identifying the patient as the exclusive source of the breakdown. This can be seen as a protective maneuver to insulate the therapist from his source of discom-

> fort—namely, the questioning of his competency, with all that this entails. . . . Once the process is recognized as evolving from a threat to self-esteem, alternative solutions to the impasse become available. Only then does the behavior which was labeled manipulative cease to be the characteristic of an unworthy patient, but an integral part of the psychopathological interactional style.

The Dependent Patient

Dependency, as a wish, may be ubiquitous, but it is encountered only occasionally as a major life theme. The length to which some patients may go to obtain dependent gratification is sometimes remarkable. For those whose wish to be cuddled or held is so intense that it resembles an addiction, sex may be used to obtain "supplies" (Hollender 1970).

Behavior that is seen or reported during the evaluation phase should alert therapists to the possibility that they are dealing with a dependent patient. Behavior that is ingratiating, compliant, and just generally too nice and too good points in that direction. Safirstein (1972) warns therapists to be on guard to avoid succumbing to patients who report just enough progress in therapy to hold the therapist's interest and to encourage the hope for a satisfying outcome. It is only when the therapist threatens to terminate the relationship that the patient's true colors are seen. As Safirstein pointed out, "It is difficult to disengage because the patient falls back on very disturbing somatic symptoms, helplessness, or suicidal threats." One subtype of the dependent patient is the so-called clinging patient who has no meaningful outside relationships and would like to turn to the therapist as the sole person in the patient's life.

Once dependent patients gain a foothold, as has been mentioned, it is extremely difficult to dislodge them. Therefore, the approach to them should be preventive. Outside relationships are to be encouraged and an intense relationship to the therapist discouraged. The latter is fostered by spacing appointments relatively far apart, limiting professional phone calls and mail, and rarely, if ever, granting requests for additional appointments.

The Needful Patient

Patients in the needful category are likely to present a story of profound deprivation in childhood. An intense craving to be held may be an important determinant of their adult behavior, and sex is bartered to obtain what they desire from a partner. Some patients are predominantly passive-dependent. Others may be slightly inappropriate in the manner in which they relate, describe physical symptoms in a bizarre fashion, and evoke a feeling of sympathy in their therapist.

The therapeutic objective with these patients is *to provide support without encouraging or promoting regression.* To accomplish this the frequency of appointments should usually be kept to once a week and the length of the session limited to 30 minutes. The reporting of dreams and fantasies should not be encouraged. The danger is that the therapist, acting on the basis of a feeling of sympathy, may increase the number and length of the visits and thereby promote regression. Moreover, when the patient does not react positively to the added attention, the therapist may feel frustrated and become resentful.

The patient's positive qualities should be recognized; making friends should be encouraged so that needs are distributed. In extreme instances, the needful patient, like the dependent patient, may become the clinging patient, and, as with the clinging patient, the chief defense for the therapist is recognizing the personality pattern and avoiding an approach which would lead to regression and incapacity. The use of a medication, mainly a low dose of a neuroleptic, may be helpful in patients who seem to have an ego defect manifested in a paranoid coloring to their reactions to close relationships.

The Powerful or Influential Patient

Some patients who are public figures have the ability to exert political or financial pressure in a variety of ways. Included are well-known entertainers, elected officials, college presidents, and top executives of large corporations. Also included in this list might be other physicians who have the capacity to influence the flow of referrals.

The referral of one of these special patients is a mixed blessing. On the positive side they tend to be interesting and they increase the therapist's sense of self-esteem. (Treating an important person makes the therapist feel more important.) On the other hand, these patients may expect or demand, through a sense of entitlement, special consideration or therapeutic procedures outside of one's ordinary practice. Often there is also added pressure to perform and to achieve a successful outcome, as illustrated by the following clinical vignette.

A college president referred a patient, described as a "major donor to this institution," to a psychiatrist on the faculty. The accompanying message was, "I want him to get the best of care," unmistakably the demand that the patient be pleased with the services provided for him.

Whether the need for a successful outcome for these patients is generated outside or comes from within, there is the danger that treatment will become more important to the therapist than to the patient. (A similar situation exists in clinics where the psychiatric resident's standing may depend to a considerable extent on the number of patients who remain in therapy.) When therapy and its outcome become overly important to the therapist, there is the increasing possibility of deviations from usual procedures. With such deviations and compromises the therapeutic process becomes progressively undermined. For example, medications not ordinarily indicated may be prescribed. With "special" patients the therapist must periodically consider whether the treatment and techniques employed are consistent with those used for other patients and, if not, then the treatment plan should be readjusted accordingly. At times a consultation with a colleague may be helpful in maintaining the correct perspective.

The Boring Patient

Periods of boredom in the practice of psychotherapy affect all psychotherapists. They may find their mind wandering, perhaps thinking ahead to lunch and a walk. Sometimes boredom becomes so intense as to induce nodding or even sleep! Many factors influence minute-to-minute enthusiasm for the psychotherapeutic process, including fatigue and concurrent personal stresses. Yet, despite these practical issues, the symptom of boredom in the therapist should serve as a possible warning signal of a countertransference problem (Altschul 1977; Morrant 1984).

Boredom may be the therapist's way of fending off material produced by the patient that might raise anxiety. For example, one therapist frequently became bored and sleepy when patients talked about their dependency needs. This was a major conflictual area for her. In supervision she learned that when she became "bored" it was a signal to pay attention to dependency issues in her patients.

Other Difficult Patients

The *entertaining patient* may succeed in engaging the therapist's attention by "playing for the audience" instead of working toward a personal goal. Here, it is essential that the therapist point out the nature of the price the patient is paying.

Offenkrantz and Tobin (1974) noted that hysterical patients may be kept in treatment after their symptoms have disappeared and treatment is no longer indicated because "they are such fun to be with."

Neill (1979), on the basis of a study he conducted, concluded that for his sample of psychiatric outpatients, the distinguishing characteristic of the difficult patient was *demanding* behavior. The *demanding patient* may be closely related to or overlap with the needful, the dependent, or the clinging patient.

Summary

Problems within the therapy or patients who become regarded as "problem patients" are an inevitable part of the psychotherapist's life. Further, there are events in therapists' lives that inevitably have an impact on psychotherapy. Similar to life itself, each of these difficult situations also represents an opportunity for therapeutic intervention and changes in the patient's usual behavior.

15

Termination of Psychotherapy

When should insight-oriented psychotherapy be terminated? Unfortunately there is no litmus-paper test, no change in color, to indicate that the endpoint has been reached. Quite the contrary, the answer to the question is highly subjective and tentative. Moreover, most treatment does not come to an end because of therapeutic considerations but, instead, is dictated by outside forces: the conclusion of residency, the relocation of the therapist or patient, or the illness or death of the therapist.

Indications for Termination

Symptom Relief

In the early days of psychoanalysis when the goal was symptom relief, it was relatively easy to decide when treatment should be terminated. But symptom relief as a goal soon proved inadequate. Jones (1936) summed up the situation as follows:

> I think we should all agree, the importance of removing symptoms is far from being the best test of therapeutic success. We know that there are endless ways in which they can be removed, that they often disappear or vary spontaneously, and that anyone who chose this as the only way of measuring the value of a therapeutic method would not be displaying much insight into the real significance of neurotic illness and would be adopting a superficial and external view of it.

Today, patients who derive relief from uncomfortable symptoms such as anxiety or depression may still regard this achievement as an indication for termination. Because motivation to continue is likely to drop off sharply, the therapist's efforts to convince the patient that further work should be done to learn more about the unconscious determinants of the symptoms usually fall short.

Character Change

When emphasis shifts from symptoms to character, the question of when to terminate therapy changed. How is it determined that the optimal type and degree of change have occurred? It is generally conceded that the therapist's goal must be realistic and as such falls far short of ideal change or cure. In attempting to establish an appropriate endpoint, several criteria were suggested. Freud (1937), while still listing relief from neurotic symptoms, added the liberation of inhibitions and abnormalities of character and the overcoming of various anxieties. Weigert (1952) mentioned the ideal of mental health, the value of maturity, and the standard of adaptation to reality. She noted, however, that these concepts are vague and ill-defined. Reich (1950) pointed out that the patient should be capable of adult object relationships, of functioning effectively at work, and of adjusting to reality.

These criteria quoted from the psychoanalytic literature and many similar ones are essentially clinical impressions, not precise measurements. Although they draw on the therapist's fund of special knowledge and experience, they are shaped largely by subjective influences. When the verbiage is stripped away, the naked facts are as follows: The therapist believes the patient is ready to terminate therapy when he or she is feeling and functioning well, or at least better than formerly, as the result of certain fundamental personality changes.

Predetermined Date

In time-limited psychotherapy and in circumstances when therapy has a built-in cutoff, a termination date is selected when the therapeutic contract is made. Consequently, the focus on termination is ever present; in a sense, the work of termination begins with the beginning of therapy. Knowing the end date in advance also makes it possible to reserve a proportionate number of hours for the terminal phase.

How Should Psychotherapy Be Terminated?

The Patient's Initiative

The subject of termination may first be broached by the patient. Mentioned initially in passing, it may be returned to for more serious consideration. On one of these occasions, the therapist might suggest that the issue be discussed more fully. It should, of course, be borne in mind that termination may be mentioned for different reasons. Under certain circumstances it is nothing more than a whim of the moment, the expression of the need to leave before bringing out feelings that might be painful to face. In this instance the patient speaks of leaving like a student thinks of quitting school right before a big examination. It is essential for the therapist to differentiate a transitory reaction, which is a *resistance*, from a more sustained reaction derived from a sense of accomplishment and a readiness to move on.

On the one hand, a patient may suddenly announce, with an air of finality, that he or she has decided to discontinue treatment. If the reasons for this decision are discussed, the impelling factors may be recognized and the decision reversed.

> However, in situations where the patient refuses to discuss the matter further, or does not keep subsequent appointments, the therapist can only accept the patient's decision. He may indicate directly or by a letter . . . his willingness to discuss the matter further if the patient elects to do so. (Dewald 1964)

On the other hand, some patients defer facing the fact that treatment is coming to an end. Orens (1955) commented,

> Although each patient, consciously at least, wants to get well and earnestly seeks the end of a successful analysis, it must always be remembered that this conscious wish may be outweighed by the unconscious satisfactions that the analysis itself may give and that this may result in a serious resistance to the end of analysis.

The danger here is that the role of being a patient in psychotherapy, like being a student in school or a patient on a medical service, may become a way of life instead of a means to an end.

The Therapist's Role

Not only should the patient's reluctance to relinquish the patient role and be separated from the therapist be noted, but the therapist's reluctance to give up the patient should also engage our attention. When two persons have worked together in a close relationship for many months or a few years, each becomes meaningful to the other. It is little wonder, then, that there is some inclination to hold on. When this inclination is intense, however, it is either an expression of a countertransference problem or of the personal use of a "captive" relationship. Fortunately, in most instances therapists are able to perceive their own tendency to hold on to patients and to overcome it.

Setting the Date

Once an agreement is reached that psychotherapy should be concluded—and this agreement may be preceded by a discussion extending over several hours—the date should be set, usually a month, six weeks, or two months off. A terminal period of this length provides time to discuss problems not previously discussed, at least not in detail, and affords the opportunity to deal with feelings of anger, grief, and separation anxiety.

Abbreviated Terminal Period

External circumstances may force an abridgement of the terminal phase. An effort should be made, however, to use the time remaining as effectively as possible to bring about some degree of closure.

> *Mrs. W's husband was being transferred to another part of the country with only two weeks' notice. Although Mrs. W had been in psychotherapy for almost a year, she expressed very little feeling about leaving. During the next to last session, she spoke on and on about the weekend she had spent with her parents and how much better she had gotten along with them.*
>
> *After twenty minutes or so, the therapist commented, "It seems to me that you are reviewing how things stand with people who are important to you. Are there feelings about therapy coming to an end that you are reluctant to talk about?" (In addition to reviewing how matters stood, Mrs. W was also reassuring herself that they were in good order.) To the therapist's comment Mrs. W responded, "Jack [her husband] asked me today, before I left to come here, how I felt. I didn't tell him." (She was also reluctant, it might be surmised, to tell the therapist and to face her feelings herself.) Mrs. W continued, "In a way this has been sort of like a crutch or something. When something bothers me I can come and talk about it." Her eyes filled with tears. As she reached for a handkerchief, she said, "And, of course, now I won't be able to." She wondered where she might turn for*

help in the future if the need arose. She also expressed the feeling that it seemed as though the therapist was leaving her instead of her leaving him. She wondered if the therapist really liked her. (If he really liked her, she suggested, he would not leave her.) During the remainder of the hour, she spoke of her feelings about termination.

Phenomena Associated with Successful Termination

At the conclusion of a course of psychotherapy, there are several common phenomena of which the therapist should be aware. Their emergence does not mean that therapy has been unsuccessful or, necessarily, that it needs be prolonged.

Mixed Feelings

Almost inevitably there will be some disappointment because treatment has not achieved all that the patient initially hoped for or expected. The expectations may have been unrealistic, somewhat like the childhood fantasy "And they lived happily ever after." One task in psychotherapy is to learn that compromises are necessary and that all pain, conflict, and tension cannot be relieved. Although further small gains might be achieved by prolonging treatment, termination is appropriate when the point of sharply diminishing returns has been reached.

Grief

The process of grief should be worked on by both patient and therapist. Psychotherapy, it should be recognized, is a genuine human relationship even if certain rules make it different from other social encounters. Each party develops genuine caring feelings about the other. Therefore, at the end there is a sense of loss to be dealt with. The patient's grief may be expressed more openly, but that of the therapist should not be underestimated or ignored.

Recrudescence of Symptoms

During the terminal phase there is often a return of the symptoms that initially brought the patient to therapy. Generally these recurrent symptoms are milder and more transient than they were originally. Several explanations have been suggested for the recrudescence of symptoms. One is that it is an unconscious expression of the wish to prolong the therapist-patient relationship. Another is that it is an expression of anxiety, a way of stating, "Look, I haven't learned enough yet; I need more time." Another possible explanation may be that it is a last effort to work through some conflicts that have not been adequately resolved. This phenomenon should not be viewed as a failure of psychotherapy, and it is not an indication for delaying termination.

Reactivation of Conflicts

Aspects of the transference relationship that previously were prominent and then appeared to recede may again become prominent. The process of termination may highlight the central issue for those patients who struggle with most conflicts about separation and loss. Because of their concerns, the transference during the terminal phase is likely to be a mother transference, and because the feelings are present in the here-and-now interpretations are much more meaningful than talking about dependency and losses in the abstract.

Separation Anxiety

The anticipation of termination often leads to an increase of anxiety similar to the anxiety a child experiences when separated from parents. It may be expressed in such terms as "I'm not sure what I can do without you" or "Who will I talk to when problems come up?" In therapy patients almost always transfer some of their dependency on their parents to the therapist. Some recurrence of anxiety in response to separation is to be expected and is not cause for special concern.

Unsuccessful Terminations

If the original goals of therapy have not been achieved when the process is brought to an end, the result can be regarded as an unsuccessful termination. Some instances are related to the therapist, others to the patient.

Therapist-Related Terminations

At times, before treatment has been successfully concluded, a variety of different circumstances may make it necessary for the therapist to terminate the therapy.

Change in professional status. Completion of training is a common reason for residents to terminate the treatment of clinic patients. If the therapist is about to leave the city, the reaction is likely to be less intense than if the therapist is to stay in the community and enter private practice. To be dropped because of an inability to pay a full fee is to be treated like a second-class citizen—a narcissistic blow that arouses anger. Even when the ground rules are clearly stated at the beginning and arrangements can be made for continued care in the clinic, the patient's feelings of abandonment may require much attention.

Illness or death. As in any interpersonal relationship, separation and loss may result from uncontrollable circumstances such as the illness or death of the therapist. The patient may react, "It's unfair" or "How can this happen to me?" Such feelings are especially prominent if a therapist commits suicide. Some patients also respond with feelings of guilt. In an infantile, omnipotent fashion, they somehow feel responsible for the circumstances that led to their abandonment.

Countertransference issues. Feelings based on the therapist's past may threaten to interfere with therapy. Such feelings might include anger at the dependent demands of the patient, a reaction of disgust in response to the patient's behavior, or sexual attraction to a patient. When the therapist recognizes that personal feelings are interfering with the therapeutic process, it would be useful to obtain the consultation of a colleague. If it is concluded that the therapist should not continue to treat the patient, it is important that the message be communicated to the patient in such a manner that the patient does not feel blame but without burdening the patient with the details of the therapist's problems.

The following vignette describes a poorly managed termination of this type.

> *A middle-aged therapist, preoccupied with his own divorce, feelings of loneliness, and financial concerns, was treating a young and attractive woman. When he began talking about his personal situation with the patient, she was interested*

and responsive. This inappropriate involvement progressed to kissing and fondling, at which point the therapist became concerned about his behavior and spoke of the need to take some action. The patient's suggestion that she transfer to another psychiatrist was not received favorably by the therapist because of his fear of being exposed. Instead, he told her that she was well and no longer needed treatment. When she eventually sought help again, the new relationship was complicated by the one with her first therapist.

Use of therapy for antitherapeutic purposes. When therapists become aware that patients are using therapy for antitherapeutic purposes, the situation should be explored actively. If, following confrontation, the behavior continues, it may be necessary to terminate treatment. In one such instance a woman used treatment and the expense of treatment as a way of punishing her husband. She repeatedly told him his behavior was the reason she required psychiatric care. When she refused to change her approach, the therapist terminated treatment, stating that when she wished to help herself rather than to punish her husband, help would be available.

Patient-Related Terminations

Patients frequently terminate therapy, sometimes so precipitously that there is little opportunity to deal with feelings or attitudes about the termination.

Move to another city. In our mobile society, patients often move. Termination under this circumstance by well-motivated patients usually presents no major difficulties. The move provides the opportunity for a review of the progress that has been made and the work that remains to be done. If there is at least time for several appointments before termination, feelings about separation can be discussed and referral made to a therapist in the patient's new location.

Financial problems. With a change in life circumstances, the patient may no longer be able to pay the therapist's regular fee. This presents a problem for both therapist and patient. A common solution is for the therapist to arrange a transfer to a low-fee clinic. Although such a move is reasonable and ethical, it does not preclude feelings of abandonment and resentment on the patient's part or guilt on the therapist's part. Clinical experiences indicate that "carrying the patient on the books" or setting up other special arrangements may make the patients feel obligated to play the role they assume their therapist expects them to play. Such was the case for a young woman who, after her divorce, could not afford the fee she had been paying. When the therapist continued to see her at a reduced fee, she felt a need to "repay" him by being the good patient and suppressing and repressing expressions of anger. On the other side of the coin, therapists may become resentful because of lost income or feelings of being used.

Intolerable emotions. As a result of the feelings elicited in psychotherapy, the patient may develop affectual states that are difficult to control or tolerate (feelings of anxiety, depression, guilt, or rage). Even the skilled therapist who attempts cautiously to titrate the amount of conflictual material elicited at any one time may occasionally discover that the patient's defenses are too fragile to integrate even relatively small amounts of affect-laden material. These patients may flee therapy, sometimes with a statement that "therapy was supposed to make me feel better, not worse."

Inability to tolerate success. Patients who are guilt-ridden and tend to be masochistic may feel that they do not deserve to be happy or successful. They are the ones who drop out of treatment at the very time that they begin to improve. This problem can be anticipated on the basis of biographical material which points to self-defeating behavior in periods of happiness and success. The pattern can sometimes be headed off or managed by anticipatory interpretations and care not to promise too much from therapy.

Devaluation of psychotherapy. Some patients, fearful of termination, seek to minimize a sense of loss by saying that therapy was not worth much anyway. These patients may tell the therapist that they derived very little and then unilaterally pick a date to terminate. Not infrequently they do not keep their last scheduled appointment.

Techniques During the Terminal Phase

The same basic principles pertain to the terminal phase as apply to earlier phases. The main difference is that the focus is on separation and loss. Various opinions have been expressed on how to conduct this phase. Several of these ideas will be presented, recognizing that certain techniques work better with some patients than with others.

"Weaning" Versus Abrupt Termination

This issue remains controversial. Some therapists believe it is helpful to "wean" the patient by scheduling appointments increasingly further apart. Others argue that weaning should not be necessary and that the process can continue unaltered to the final session.

Trial Terminations

Alexander and French (1946) suggested that periodic vacations or trial terminations are an effective way of determining how well the goals of therapy have been met. Patients can recognize the areas in need of further attention and are likely to return to treatment with a strong motivation to change.

Offers of Future Help

The offer of future help if needed carries with it a double message. For some patients it means that further difficulties are expected, whereas for others it is reassuring to know the therapist is willing to be of assistance. Neither the patient nor the therapist should have the illusion that future problems will not occur. Life circumstances change, and at times old defensive patterns may recur or new problems may appear. The patient should be able to handle most situations alone. For the occasional problem requiring additional assistance, an hour or two with the therapist will often prove adequate.

Avoiding Confrontation

It is not unusual for patients to decide that they are ready to terminate therapy at a time when the therapist thinks otherwise. The therapist may state his or her opinion but should not take an inflexible stand. The way should be left open for the patient to return at a later date or pursue therapy with another therapist.

Transfers to a New Therapist

When a transfer occurs, a variety of emotions are evoked on the part of both the patient and the therapist. If the patient feels abandoned or rejected, angry feelings may be displaced to the new therapist. It is unfortunate if the two therapists are openly competitive with each other. For the best interest of the patient, the positive aspects of having a new therapist should be emphasized. Not only should the first therapist express a positive regard for the professional qualifications of the new therapist, but the original therapist should also underscore the fact that it may be helpful to have a fresh perspective on the patient's problems.

The Ending

As Buxbaum (1950) stated, "The termination of the analysis is an important phase of therapy. It is like the finale in a musical movement which repeats the leading motives of the piece." During the final hours the patients may attempt to summarize what has been accomplished. Not infrequently they will conclude that much has been accomplished—not everything, but enough—and that to remain in therapy longer would be neither helpful nor desirable. To be sure, patients may vacillate, but it is hoped that the self-assured attitude will prevail.

During the final hour there is usually a discussion of what lies ahead. Patients can be reminded or they may remind themselves that after the "course work" is concluded, they can still "pursue studies" on their own when they are so inclined or feel the need.

Often patients will express their gratitude for the help they have received. At such a time—usually during the last few minutes of the final hour—the therapist may respond by stating that he or she has enjoyed working with the patient if such has been the case. This exchange ends the relationship on an appropriate note—each acknowledging the fact that something positive has been derived from the other.

Termination of Supportive Psychotherapy

Although some of the statements made about a terminal phase for insight-oriented psychotherapy might apply to supportive psychotherapy, many do not. Moreover, the use of a technique referred to as "spacing and spanning" is particularly applicable to patients in supportive psychotherapy. By spacing and spanning is meant gradually increasing the length of time between appointments geared to the patient's tolerance. When the time interval has become great, the next step is to eliminate any set time and operate on a "prn" (as needed) basis. In other words, patients on this schedule will be seen only when they call for appointments. If the pacing has been good and outside circumstances remain relatively stable, calls will be infrequent, perhaps once or twice a year or even less often.

Summary

Termination is an important part of the therapeutic process. Rather than regarding it as a tack-on to the end of psychotherapy, it should be a phase anticipated throughout the entire course of treatment. At times, it is highlighted by setting a termination date early in the therapy. With patients whose major problems stem from issues related to loss and separation or dependency versus autonomy, a substantial part of the therapeutic work is accomplished during the latter part of therapy and the terminal phase.

References

Alexander FG: The relation of structural and instinctual conflicts. Psychoanal Q 2:181–207, 1933

Alexander F, French TM: Psychoanalytic Therapy: Principles and Application. New York, The Ronald Press Company, 1946

Allport GW: Pattern and Growth in Personality. New York, Holt, Rinehart and Winston, 1961

Altschul VA: The so-called boring patient. Am J Psychiatry 31:533–545, 1977

American Psychiatric Association: Diagnostic and Statistical Manual of Mental Disorders, 3rd Ed, Revised. Washington, DC, American Psychiatric Association, 1987

Ballenger JC: Pharmacotherapy of the panic disorders. J Clin Psychiatry 47(Suppl):27–32, 1986

Barhash AZ: Psychiatric techniques in medical practice. JAMA 146: 1584–1588, 1951

Bellak L: Once over: what is psychotherapy? J Nerv Ment Dis 165:295–299, 1977

Budman SH, Stone J: Advances in brief psychotherapy: a review of recent literature. Hosp Community Psychiatry 34:939–946, 1983

Buxbaum E: The technique of terminating analysis. Int J Psychoanal 31:184–190, 1950

Castelnuovo-Tedesco P: The Twenty-Minute Hour: A Guide to Brief Psychotherapy for the Physician. Boston, Little, Brown, 1965 [paperback reprint edition: Washington, DC, American Psychiatric Press]

Cloninger CR: A systematic method for clinical description and classification of personality variables. Arch Gen Psychiatry 44:573–588, 1987

Colby KM: A Primer for Psychotherapists. New York, Ronald Press Company, 1951

Conte HR, Plutchik R: Controlled research in supportive psychotherapy. Psychiatric Annals 16:530–533, 1986

Conte HR, Plutchik R, Wild KR, et al: Combined psychotherapy and pharmacotherapy for depression. Arch Gen Psychiatry 43:471–479, 1986

Cooper AM: Will neurobiology influence psychoanalysis? Am J Psychiatry 142:1395–1402, 1985

Davanloo H: Techniques of short-term dynamic psychotherapy. Psychiatr Clin North Am 2:11–22, 1979

Deutsch F: The associative anamesis. Psychoanal Q 8:354–381, 1939

Devereux G: Some criteria for the timing of confrontations and interpretations. Int J Psychoanal 32:19–24, 1951

Dewald PA: Psychotherapy: A Dynamic Approach. New York, Basic Books, 1964

Docherty SP, Fiester SJ: The therapeutic alliance and compliance with psychopharmacology, in Psychiatry Update: American Psychiatric Association Annual Review, Volume 4. Edited by Hales RE, Frances AJ. Washington, DC, American Psychiatric Press, 1985, pp 607–632

Eissler KR: The effect of the structure of the ego on psychoanalytic technique. J Am Psychoanal Assoc 1:104–143, 1953

Elkin I, Shea MT, Watkins JT, et al: National Institute of Mental Health treatment of depression collaborative research program: general effectiveness of treatments. Arch Gen Psychiatry 46: 971–982, 1989

Fenichel O: Problems of Psychoanalytic Technique. Albany, NY, The Psychoanalytic Quarterly, 1941

Fenichel O: The Psychoanalytic Theory of Neurosis. New York, W.W. Norton, 1945

Frances A, Perry S: Transference interpretations in focal therapy. Am J Psychiatry 140:405–409, 1983

Frank JD: The dynamics of the psychotherapeutic relationship: determinants and effects of the therapist's influence. Psychiatry 22:17–39, 1959

Frank JD: Therapeutic factors in psychotherapy. Am J Psychother 25:350–361, 1971

French TM: The transference phenomenon, in Psychoanalytic Therapy. Edited by Alexander F, French TM. New York, Ronald Press, 1946, pp 71–95

French TM: The art and science of psychoanalysis. J Am Psychoanal Assoc 6:197–214, 1958

Freud A: The Ego and Mechanisms of Defense. New York, International Universities Press, 1936

Freud S: The interpretation of dreams (1900), in The Standard Edition of the Complete Psychological Works of Sigmund Freud, Vol IV and V. Translated and edited by Strachey J. London, Hogarth Press, 1953, pp 1–621

Freud S: Fragment of an analysis of a case of hysteria (1905a), in The Standard Edition of the Complete Psychological Works of Sigmund Freud, Vol VII. Translated and edited by Strachey J. London, Hogarth Press, 1953, pp 7–122

Freud S: On psychotherapy (1905b), in The Standard Edition of the Complete Psychological Works of Sigmund Freud, Vol VII. Translated and edited by Strachey J. London, Hogarth Press, 1953, pp 257–268

Freud S: Notes upon a case of obsessional neurosis (1909), in The Standard Edition of the Complete Psychological Works of Sigmund Freud, Vol X. Translated and edited by Strachey J. London, Hogarth Press, 1955, pp 159–249

Freud S: Recommendations to physicians practicing psychoanalysis (1912), in The Standard Edition of the Complete Psychological Works of Sigmund Freud, Vol XII. Translated and edited by Strachey J. London, Hogarth Press, 1958, pp 111–120

Freud S: On beginning the treatment (further recommendations on the technique of psychoanalysis) (1913), in The Standard Edition of the Complete Psychological Works of Sigmund Freud, Vol XII. Translated and edited by Strachey J. London, Hogarth Press, 1958, pp 123–144

Freud S: Analysis terminal and interminable (1937), in The Standard Edition of the Complete Psychological Works of Sigmund Freud, Vol XXIII. Translated and edited by Strachey J. London, Hogarth Press, 1964, pp 209–253

Freud S: An outline of psychoanalysis (1940) [1938], in The Standard Edition of the Complete Psychological Works of Sigmund Freud, Vol XXIII. Translated and edited by Strachey J. London, Hogarth Press, 1974, pp 144–207

Gitelson M: Psychoanalysis and dynamic psychiatry. AMA Archives of Neurology and Psychiatry 66:280–288, 1951

Greenbaum H: Psychoanalyst's evolution from orthodoxy to heterodoxy. Academy Forum 30:3–6, 1986

Greenson RR: On the silence and sounds of the analytic hour. J Am Psychoanal Assoc 9:79–84, 1961

Greenson RR: Beyond transference and interpretation. Int J Psychoanal 53:213–217, 1972

Greenson RR, Wexler M: The non-transference relationship in the psychoanalytic situation. Int J Psychoanal 50:27–39, 1969

Group for the Advancement of Psychiatry: Pharmacotherapy and Psychotherapy: Paradoxes, Problems, and Progress. Report No. 93. GAP Report Series 9:261–431, 1975

Halleck SL: The Treatment of Emotional Disorders. New York, Aronson, 1978

Heimann P: On counter-transference. Int J Psychoanal 31:81–84, 1950

Henderson LJ: Physician and patient as a social system. N Engl J Med 212:819–823, 1935

Hollender MH: Ambulatory schizophrenia. J Chronic Dis 9:249–259, 1959

Hollender MH: Is the wish to sleep a universal motive for dreaming? J Am Psychoanal Assoc 10:323–328, 1962

Hollender MH: The Practice of Psychoanalytic Psychotherapy. New York, Grune and Stratton, 1965

Hollender MH: The need or wish to be held. Arch Gen Psychiatry 22:445–453, 1970

Hollender MH: Psychiatry's sacred cows (editorial). J Clin Psychiatry 40:158, 1979

Hollender MH: The case of Anna O: a reformulation. Am J Psychiatry 137:797–800, 1980

Hollender MH, Shevitz S: The seductive patient. South Med J 71:776–779, 1978

Hollingshead AB, Redlich FC: Social Class and Mental Illness: A Community Study. New York, John Wiley and Sons, 1958

Holt RR: The current status of psychoanalytic theory. Psychoanalytic Psychology 2:289–315, 1985

Horney K: Neurosis and Human Growth. New York, W.W. Norton, 1950

Jones E: The criteria of success in treatment (1936), in Papers on Psychoanalysis, 5th Ed. Baltimore, Williams and Wilkins, 1948

Jones E: The Life and Work of Sigmund Freud, Vol I. New York, Basic Books, 1953

Karasu TB: General principles of psychotherapy in specialized techniques, in Individual Psychotherapy. Edited by Karasu TB, Bellak L. New York, Brunner/Mazel, 1980

Karasu TB: Psychotherapy and pharmacotherapy: toward an integrative model. Am J Psychiatry 139:1102–1113, 1982

Karasu TB: The specificity version nonspecialty dilemma: toward identifying therapeutic change agents. Am J Psychiatry 143: 687–695, 1986

Klerman GL, Budman S, Berwick D, et al: Efficacy of a brief psychosocial intervention for symptoms of stress and distress among patients in primary care. Med Care 25:1078–1088, 1987

Krasner L: Studies of the conditioning of verbal behavior. Psychol Bull 55:148–170, 1958

Krystal H: Alexithymia and psychotherapy. Am J Psychother 33:17–31, 1979

Langer SK: Philosophy in a New Key: A Study in the Symbolism of Reason, Rite, and Art. New York, Mentor Books, 1942

Leslie A: Lady Randolph Churchill. New York, Lancer Books, 1969, pp 219–222

Levine M: Psychotherapy in Medical Practice. New York, Macmillan, 1947

Lewin KK: Nonverbal cues and transference. Arch Gen Psychiatry 12:391–394, 1965

Lisansky ET: Roundtable: dealing with the seductive patient. Medical Aspects of Human Sexuality 10:97, 1976

Macalpine I: The development of the transference. Psychoanal Q 19:501–539, 1950

Mackenzie TB, Rosenberg SD, Bergen BJ, et al: The manipulative patient: an interactional approach. Psychiatry 41:264–271, 1978

Malan DH: Toward the Validation of Dynamic Psychotherapy. New York, Plenum, 1980

Mandler G, Kaplan WK: Subjective evaluation and reinforcing effect of a verbal stimulus. Science 124:582–583, 1956

Mann J: Time-Limited Psychotherapy. Cambridge, Mass, Harvard University Press, 1973

Marmor J: A re-evaluation of certain aspects of psychoanalytic theory and practice, in Modern Concept of Psychoanalysis. Edited by Salzman J, Masserman JH. New York, Philosophical Library, 1962

Marmor J: Short-term dynamic psychotherapy. Am J Psychiatry 136:149–155, 1979

Menninger K: Theory of Psychoanalytic Technique. New York, Science Editions, 1961

Michels R: Treatment of the difficult patient in psychotherapy. Canadian Psychiatric Association Journal 22:117–121, 1977

Miller MH: The borderline psychotic patient: the importance of diagnosis in medical and surgical practice. Ann Intern Med 46:736–743, 1957

Morrant JCA: Boredom in psychiatric practice. Canadian J Psychiatry 29:431–434, 1984

Nadelson C, Notman M, Arons E, et al: The pregnant therapist. Am J Psychiatry 131:1107–1111, 1974

Neill J: The difficult patient: identification and response. J Clin Psychiatry 40:209–212, 1979

Offenkrantz W, Tobin A: Psychoanalytic psychotherapy. Arch Gen Psychiatry 30:593–606, 1974

Orens MH: Setting a termination date: an impetus to analysis. J Am Psychoanal Assoc 3:651–665, 1955

Perry S, Cooper AM, Michels R: The psychodynamic formulation: its purpose, structure, and clinical application. Am J Psychiatry 144:543–550, 1987

Pine F: Supportive psychotherapy: a psychoanalytic perspective. Psychiatric Annals 16:526–529, 1986

Rappaport EA: Beyond traumatic neurosis. Int J Psychoanal 49:719–731, 1968

Reich A: On the termination of analysis. Int J Psychoanal 31:179–183, 1950

Reich A: On counter-transference. Int J Psychoanal 32:25–31, 1951

Reiser MF: Are psychiatric educators "losing the mind"? Am J Psychiatry 145:148–153, 1988

Robertiello RC, Schoenewolf G: One Hundred and One Common Therapeutic Errors: Countertransference and Counterresistance in Psychotherapy. New York, Aronson, 1987

Sabshin M, Ramot J: Pharmacotherapeutic evaluation and the psychiatric setting. AMA Archives of Neurology and Psychiatry 75:362–370, 1956

Safirstein SL: The clinging patient: a serious management problem. Canadian Psychiatric Association Journal 17:SS221–SS225, 1972

Shapiro ET, Pinsker H: Shared ethnic scotoma. Am J Psychiatry 130:1338–1341, 1973

Sifneos P: Short-Term Psychotherapy and Emotional Crisis. Cambridge, Mass, Harvard University Press, 1972

Sifneos P: The current status of individual short-term dynamic psychotherapy and its future: an overview. Am J Psychother 38:472–483, 1984

Sim M: Management and medical practice (letter). Am J Psychiatry 138:1512, 1981

Spitz RA: Transference: the analytic setting and its prototype. Int J Psychoanal 37:380–385, 1956

Strupp HH: Toward a specification of teaching and learning in psychotherapy. Arch Gen Psychiatry 21:203–212, 1969

Strupp HH: On the technology of psychotherapy. Arch Gen Psychiatry 26:270–278, 1972

Strupp HH: On the basic ingredients of psychotherapy. J Consult Clin Psychol 41:1–8, 1973

Strupp HH: The nonspecific hypothesis of therapeutic effectiveness: a current assessment. Am J Orthopsychiatry 56:513–552, 1986

Strupp HH, Binder JL: Psychotherapy in a New Key: A Guide to Time-Limited Dynamic Psychotherapy. New York, Basic Books, 1986

Strupp HH, Hadley SW: Specific vs. nonspecific factors in psychotherapy. Arch Gen Psychiatry 36:1125–1136, 1979

Strupp HH, Hadley SW, Gomes-Schwartz B: Psychotherapy for Better or Worse: The Problem of Negative Effects. New York, Aronson, 1977

Sullivan HS: The psychiatric interview, in The Psychiatric Interview. Edited by Perry HS, Gawel ML. New York, W.W. Norton, 1954, pp 99–101

Szasz TS: On the experience of the analyst in the psychoanalytic situation: a contribution to the theory of psychoanalytic treatment. J Am Psychoanal Assoc 4:197–223, 1956

Szasz TS, Hollender MH: A contribution to the philosophy of medicine: the basic models of the doctor-patient relationship. AMA Archives of Internal Medicine 97:585–592, 1956

Tower LE: Countertransference. J Am Psychoanal Assoc 4:224–255, 1956

Tseng WS, McDermott JF Jr: Psychotherapy, historical roots, universal elements, and cultural variations. Am J Psychiatry 132:378–384, 1975

Vaillant G, Bond M, Vaillant CO: An empirically validated hierarchy of defense mechanisms. Arch Gen Psychiatry 45:786–794, 1986

Waelder R: Introduction to the discussion on problems of transference. Int J Psychoanal 37:367–368, 1956

Wahl CW: The technique of brief psychotherapy with hospitalized psychosomatic patients. International Journal of Psychoanalytic Psychotherapy 1:69–82, 1972

Waterhouse GJ, Strupp HH: The patient-therapist relationship: research from the psychodynamic perspective. Clinical Psychology Review 4:77–92, 1984

Webb WL: Ethics and psychiatry, in The American Psychiatric Press Textbook of Psychiatry. Edited by Talbott JA, Hales RE,

Yudofsky SC. Washington, DC, American Psychiatric Press, 1988, pp 1085–1096

Weigert E: Contribution to the problem of terminating psychoanalyses. Psychoanal Q 21:465–480, 1952

Weissberg JH: Short-term dynamic psychotherapy: an application of psychoanalytic personality theory. J Am Acad Psychoanal 12: 101–113, 1984

Wolberg LR: The Technique of Psychotherapy. New York, Grune and Stratton, 1954

Wolberg LR: The technique of short-term psychotherapy, in Short-Term Psychotherapy. Edited by Wolberg LR. New York, Grune and Stratton, 1965, pp 177–200

Wolf S, Pinsky RH: Effects of placebo administration and occurrence of toxic reactions. JAMA 155:339–341, 1954

Wolstein B: Transference, 2nd ed. New York, Grune and Stratton, 1964

Woody GE, McLellan AT, Luborsky L, et al: Twelve-month follow-up of psychotherapy for opiate dependence. Am J Psychiatry 144:590–596, 1987

Name Index

Subject Index